The Essential
Air Fryer Cookbook

675 Foolproof, Quick & Amazingly Easy Air Fryer Recipes For Beginners and Advanced Users

Jennifer William

Text Copyright © Jennifer William

All rights reserved. No part of this guide may be reproduced in any form without permission in writing from the publisher except in the case of brief quotations embodied in critical articles or reviews.

Legal & Disclaimer

The information contained in this book and its contents is not designed to replace or take the place of any form of medical or professional advice; and is not meant to replace the need for independent medical, financial, legal or other professional advice or services, as may be required. The content and information in this book has been provided for educational and entertainment purposes only.

The content and information contained in this book has been compiled from sources deemed reliable, and it is accurate to the best of the Author's knowledge, information and belief. However, the Author cannot guarantee its accuracy and validity and cannot be held liable for any errors and/or omissions. Further, changes are periodically made to this book as and when needed. Where appropriate and/or necessary, you must consult a professional (including but not limited to your doctor, attorney, financial advisor or such other professional advisor) before using any of the suggested remedies, techniques, or information in this book.

Upon using the contents and information contained in this book, you agree to hold harmless the Author from and against any damages, costs, and expenses, including any legal fees potentially resulting from the application of any of the information provided by this book. This disclaimer applies to any loss, damages or injury caused by the use and application, whether directly or indirectly, of any advice or information presented, whether for breach of contract, tort, negligence, personal injury, criminal intent, or under any other cause of action.

Contents

Introduction **6**

Chapter 1: Introduction to the Air Fryer **7**
    How does it work? 7
    Why use Air Fryers 7
    Tips for Using Your Air Fryer 8

Chapter 2: Air Fryer Tasty Breakfast Recipes **9**
    Oatmeal Bread In The Fryer 9
    Potato Bread 10
    Bauru 11
    Cheese Bread 12
    Mini Croissant 13
    Bread With Sausage 14
    Australian Bread (Outback Style) 15
    Rustic potato 16
    Onion Stuffed With Ricotta 17
    Tomato Stuffed With Moroccan Couscous 19
    Delicious Garlic Bread 20
    Crispy Vegetables 21
    Rustic Sweet Potatoes Without Frying 22
    Tuna And Sweet Potato 23
    Tapioca Dadinho 24
    Australian Gluten Free Bread 25
    Damper 26
    Leaf Bread 27
    French Cheese Fries 28
    Pizza With Homemade Dough 29
    Bread With Egg 30
    Australian Panettone 31
    Puff Pastry 32
    Fried Egg 33
    Mexican Lentils 34

Chapter 3: Air Fryer Snacks and Appetizers **35**
    Anzac Cookie 35
    Apple Pie Australian 36
    Greek Barbecue/Kebab 37
    Roasted Peanuts 38
    Banana Chips 39
    Fugazza 40
    Antipasto 41
    Mozzarella Sticks 42
    Portuguese Chestnut 44
    Cassava Dumpling With Dried Meat Filling 45

    Kibbeh Fried 47
    Rain Balls 48
    Rolls Ham And Cheese 49
    Rice Balls 50
    Patty 51
    Bolovo 52
    Conservation Of Cod In Italian Bread 53
    Crutones 54
    Tomato And Cheese Bruschetta 55
    American Rosca Recipe 56
    Granola Cookies 57
    Banana Cookies 58
    Pizza Fit 59
    Bread Cake 60
    Onion Rings In Beer 61
    Bread With Pepper And Garlic Confit 62
    Cocoa Bread 63
    Quick Banana Bread 64
    Pullman Bread 65
    Onion Cream On Italian Bread 66
    Pecan Pie With Breadcrumbs 67
    Bread Cake With Apples And Dried Figs 68
    Fried Yucca 69
    Fried Plantain 70
    Baked Cheese Bread 71
    Heart Of Palm Balls 72
    Breaded Camembert Cheese 73
    Rye And Chorizo Bread 74
    Sweet Fried Potatoes 75
    Crispy Ham And Cheese Patty 76
    Pumpkin Cream On Italian Bread 77
    Spring Roll 78
    Palmetto 79
    Croque Monsieur 80
    Bread Gnocchi 81

Chapter 4: Air Fryer Poultry Recipes **82**
    Chicken Meatballs 82
    Homemade Breaded Nugget In Doritos 83
    Chicken Breast 84
    Homemade Chicken Nuggets 85
    Breaded Chicken Without Flour 86
    Buffalo Wings 87
    Barbecue With Chorizo and Chicken 88
    Roasted Thigh 89
    Hot Smoked Wings 90
    Coxinha Fit 91
    Rolled Turkey Breast 92

Chicken In Beer 93
Chicken Fillet 94
Chicken Thigh With Potatoes 95
Chicken Wings With Mustard 96
Chicken With Lemon And Bahian Seasoning 97
Whole Chicken 98
Chicken Fingers 99

Chapter 5: Air Fryer Meat (Beef, Pork and Lamb) Recipes 100

Interior Pork Rib 100
Elegant Interior Ribs 102
Stuffed Loin 103
Kafta 104
Pork Tenderloin With Mustard And Honey 105
Picanha In Bread Bag 106
Meatballs 107
Breaded Suckling Pig Fillet 108
Milanese Steak 109
Pork Rind 110
Barbecue Picanha 111
Greek Barbecue 112
Barbecue With Skewers 113
Barbecue With Homemade Kafta 114
Breaded Steak 115
Pork Fillet Medallions 116
Beef Parmigiana 117
Meat With Rustic Potatoes 118
Pumpkin With Beef 119
Filet Mignon With Gorgonzola Sauce 120
Meat In Wine Sauce 121

Chapter 6: Seafood Recipes 122

Fried Manjubinha 122
Kanikama Stick 123
Light Fried Fish 124
SHRIMP 125
Cod 126
Breaded Fillet Of Hake 127
Fish Bait 128
Tilapia Fillet 129
Tilapia on Papillot 130
Coconut Breaded Shrimp 131
Salmon With Orange Sauce 132
Cod With Breadcrumbs 133
Fried Squid 134
Fish With Vegetables 135
Sardine Pizza 136
Cod With Capers 137
Tilapia With Mushrooms And Paprika ... 138
Tilapia With Sweet Potatoes 139

Chapter 7: Air Fryer Vegetables Recipes 140

Lentil Dumpling 140
Risotto Balls 142
Fried Soybeans 143
Brazilian Pine Nuts 144
Breadcrumbs With Dried Fruit 145
Eggplant Paste 146
Cereal Bar 147
Fried Capeletti 148
Caponata With Aubergines And Zucchini 149
Spinach Balls 150
Quick Vegetable Pie 151
Vegetables With Herbs 152
Assorted Vegetables 153
5 Roasted Vegetables 154
Roasted Zucchini 155
Carrot Roasted 156
Vegetables With Coconut Oil 157
Roasted Eggplant 158
Fried Chickpeas 159
Eggplant lasagna 160
Vegetable Mix 161
Eggplant Sticks 162

Chapter 8: Air Fryer Dessert Recipes 163

Australian Chocolate Pie 163
Australian Brownie 165
Angu Cake 166
Cake With Homemade Dough 168
Italian Style Coffee Cake 170
Bean Stew Cookie 171
Chicken Meat Patty 172
Rolled Pizza 173
Hot Dog 175
Stuffed Cauliflower 176
Sequilho 178
Fried Polenta 179
Churros Filled With Caramel 181
Bisnaguinha Gluten Free Bread 182
Salty French Toast 183
Sausage Braid 184
Super Burger 185
Soufflé 187
Pine Nut Balls 188

Blender cake 189	Bread Lasagna And White Sauce 210
Zucchini Soufflé With Cheese And Ham 190	Portuguese Flatbread Pizza 211
Hot Canape 191	Zucchini Bolognese Lasagna 212
Cheese Fondue 192	Margherita Pizza 213
Lasagna 193	Banana Cake 214
Amazing Condensed Milk Pudding 194	S'mores 215
American Toast With Fried Egg In The Middle 196	Rosca de Polvilho 216
Fried Aubergine Breading A Milanesa 197	Banana Covered-Soft Paste 217
Homemade French Toast 198	Coconut Tartlets 218
Coffee Cake 199	Honey Bread Buns 219
Chocolate Molten Lava Cake 200	Herbs Bread 220
Petit Gateau 202	Cheesecake 221
Sweet Cookie With Coco 203	Lemon Cake 222
Sweet Corn Cake With Guava Pasta 205	
Layered Apple Pie 206	
Tortilla Caprese 207	
German Garlic Bread 208	
Wholemeal Bread With Egg Curry 209	

Conclusion 224

Introduction

Eating healthy depends not only on the type of food consumed, but on many other factors, such as how you cook and the time it takes you to prepare your favorite dish. In other words, many habits and customs that are followed when it comes to eating play an important role in maintaining good health.

While healthy diet consists of eating a variety of foods that provide you with the nutrients you need to stay healthy, feel good and have energy; many ways of cooking make us lose the nutrients which include protein, carbohydrates, fats, water, vitamins, and minerals.

For this reason, they invent the appliances such as Air Fryer. With this appliance, you can cook what you want without taking too long while your food does not lose any nutrient. So, in this book, you will find, not only tips for using Air Fryer, but also some tasty recipes for breakfast, snacks and appetizers, poultry, meat (Beef, Pork and Lamb), vegetables and desserts that will help you save your time, but also to eating in a healthy way.

Enjoy it!!

Chapter 1

Introduction to the Air Fryer

The air fryer circulates hot air around the food. This allows the result to be crispy on the outside and soft on the inside and, of course, just as tasty as a traditional fry, without the heaviness and consumption of fats that are harmful to health. Air fryers allow food to cook up to 30% faster. The innovative technology is very easy to clean and incredibly durable.

How does it work?

The air fryers, in general terms, work thanks to hot air, which circulates around the food container and cooks it little by little. Thanks to the electric current, the air that comes out through the air vents cooks the food in much the same way as oil fryers, leaving the outside very crisp.

The truth is that these types of oil-free deep fryers are great for all those who want to enjoy delicious potatoes, dumplings or breaded chicken strips without the need for them to be full of fat, without a doubt, a much healthier option.

Why use Air Fryers

In addition to being a healthier way to eat (the biggest advantage of these fryers) another of the advantages of hot air fryers is that they are much cleaner, in two ways. On the one hand you will not have to worry about the oil leaping and staining the counter, nor will it leave a fried smell throughout the house.

On the other hand, they are very easy to clean. There are many models of this type of fryer that can be placed directly in the dishwasher. In any case, even when washed by hand, they are infinitely easier and faster to clean, since we will not have to make an effort to remove the grease from the oil.

Finally, the advantage that seems most convincing to many of us is that this type of hot air fryer will also save you a lot of money. By having to invest only a tablespoon of oil, you will consume less and, without a doubt, you will see how your oil bottles will last you much longer.

Tips for Using Your Air Fryer

<u>Always have the rack in the basket</u>

This allows hot air to circulate around the food and also prevents food from settling in excess oil.

<u>Deep fryers are noisy</u>. When it is running, you will hear buzzing from fans.

<u>It's practical</u>. Even browning requires you to remove the basket and mix the food every few minutes.

<u>It's okay to take out the basket to take a look</u>

You can do this at any point in the cooking process. There is no need to turn off the machine as it turns itself off when the basket is out.

<u>Make sure the drawer is fully inserted or it will not turn back on</u>

You will know, because the air fryer will suddenly be silent.

Food cooks fast, faster than you're used to! It is one of the best attributes of the fryer. The manual for your air fryer probably has a useful table of cooking times and temperatures for common foods. The less food there is in the basket, the shorter the cooking time will be. The more food, the longer it will be.

<u>You may need a slightly lower temperature</u>

Many recipes for air fryers require lower temperature settings than their conventional counterparts. This may seem suspicious, but go with it. Again, fryers heat up very quickly and move that hot air, so a slightly lower temperature will help prevent food from accumulating. also dark or crispy on the outside, while cooking properly on the inside.

<u>Do not grease the drawer with spray oil</u>

It seems like it would be a good idea, right? But the baskets have a non-stick coating, and the cooking spray can damage the finish over time. (Actually, it says so in the manual! What, didn't you read it?)

Instead of cooking spray, mix the food with oil, you're probably already doing it, in many cases, or rub it with an oil-saturated paper towel. I discovered that previously fried frozen foods did not need the help of extra fat.

<u>Don't clutter the drawer</u>

Because of all the space they take up on a countertop, deep fryers don't have a large capacity. For best results, don't load the drawer with food (the image used in fryer marketing is quite misleading). It is very tempting to add another handful of shaved potato or beet sticks, but you will learn from experience that food comes out crispier and cooks faster if you work in small batches.

Chapter 2

Air Fryer Tasty Breakfast Recipes

Oatmeal Bread In The Fryer

Servings: 2
Preparation time: 5 minutes
Cook time: 25 minutes

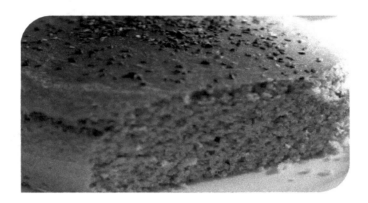

Ingredients

- 1 ¼ cup warm milk
- ¼ cup olive oil or olive oil
- 1 sachet of dry organic yeast
- ¼ cup sugar
- 2 eggs
- 1 ½ cup all-purpose flour
- 1 ½ cup oat bran
- 1 tsp salt

Steps to Cook

1. Mix warm milk well with olive oil, yeast, sugar and eggs.
2. Add the flour, bran and salt and mix until it turns into a kind of porridge
3. Place the dough in a greased and floured skillet that will fit in the fryer.
4. Bake for 10 minutes at 176°F.
5. After that time, increase to 320°F and bake for another 15 minutes.
6. Serve with a cup of tea or coffee.

Nutrition Information

- Calories: 71
- Carbohydrates: 12.3g
- Fat: 1.1g
- Protein: 2.2g
- Sugar: 11g
- Cholesterol: 0mg

Potato Bread

Servings: 4
Preparation time: 60 minutes
Cook time: 10 minutes

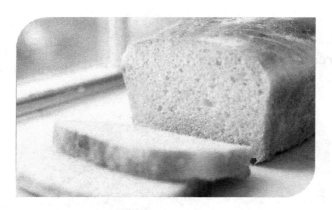

Ingredients

- 1 cup warm milk with 1 egg inside
- ½ cup instant mashed potatoes + ½ cup water
- 2 tbsp butter or margarine
- 1 tbsp of olive oil or olive oil
- 1 ½ tbsp of salt
- 2 tbsp of sugar
- 3 cups of flour
- 2 ½ tsp of dry organic yeast
- 1 egg yolk to brush

Steps to Cook

1. Put all the ingredients in a bowl, mix and knead well until you get smooth and very soft dough.
2. If you have a bread machine, put all the ingredients in the bread machine shape and set the kneading or dough cycle and let it beat for at least 30 minutes.
3. With the dough ready, divide it into 16 equal parts and make a ball with each piece of dough.
4. If you are filling just flatten the dough in the palm of your hand, then put the filling of your choice and close by joining the edges to the center, then rotate and place on a baking sheet greased with oil or olive oil, repeat the process with all the balls, then brush with egg yolk and let it rest, covered with plastic wrap or in a plastic bag, for 20 to 30 minutes.
5. Place 4 potato rolls at a time in the Air Fryer basket and adjust for 10 minutes at 350°F.

Nutrition Information

- Calories: 100
- Carbohydrates: 20g
- Fat: 1g
- Protein: 4g
- Sugar: 4g
- Cholesterol: 0mg

Bauru

Servings: 4
Preparation time: 30 minutes
Cook time: 15 minutes

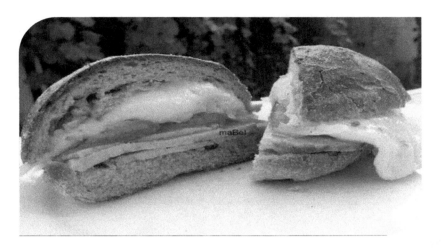

Ingredients

- 2 ¼ lb of sour sparks
- 1 tbsp of salt
- ½ American glass of boiling water
- ½ lb margarine
- 4 eggs
- 2 cups of milk
- ½ lb grated Minas cheese

Steps to Cook

2. Whisk all the ingredients of the dough in the blender, first the liquids.
3. After choosing the filling, grease the plate that you are going to put into the fryer and flour, place a layer of dough, a layer of filling and cover with another layer of dough.
4. Put in the air fryer at 350°F for about 45 minutes.

Nutrition Information

- Calories: 350
- Carbohydrates: 40g
- Fat: 5g
- Protein: 6g
- Sugar: 5g
- Cholesterol: 300mg

Cheese Bread

Servings: 4
Preparation time: 30 minutes
Cook time: 15 minutes

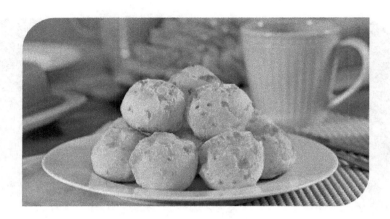

Ingredients

- 3 eggs
- ½ cup of oil
- 1 cup milk
- 2 cups flour
- ½ cup of cottage cheese
- 1 small tsp of salt
- 1 large tbsp of baking powder

Steps to Cook

6. Mix the salt with the starch in a bowl. While stirring, add the boiling water little by little. Then add the eggs, margarine, milk and stir. When a homogeneous mass remains, add the grated cheese and knead well, until the mass is uniform and loosens from the hands.
7. Roll the dough into balls and place on a baking sheet and freeze.
8. Place the balls in the basket of your fryer 1 cm away. Adjust the Air fryer for 15 minutes at 390°F. Check before time runs out.
9. Serve with a cup of tea or coffee.

Nutrition Information

- Calories: 100
- Carbohydrates: 20g
- Fat: 1g
- Protein: 4g
- Sugar: 4g
- Cholesterol: 0mg

Mini Croissant

Servings: 2
Preparation time: 10 minutes
Cook time: 15 minutes

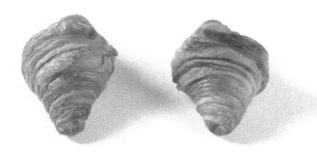

Ingredients

- Puff pastry
- Filling of your choice
- Egg (clear and separate yolk)

Steps to Cook

1. Open the puff pastry on a flat, smooth surface, cut into triangles, then take each triangle and place the chosen filling on the widest end.
2. Brush the egg whites over the edge of the dough and roll up, squeeze the ends a little to close tightly.
3. After shaping all of them, brush with egg yolks on top and sprinkle sesame, seeds or grated cheese.
4. Place the croissants in the basket of the Air Fryer and adjust for 15 minutes at 390°F.

Nutrition Information

- Calories: 114
- Carbohydrates: 13g
- Fat: 5.9g
- Protein: 2.3g
- Sugar: 3.2g
- Cholesterol: 19mg

Bread With Sausage

Servings: 2
Preparation time: 5 minutes
Cook time: 10 minutes

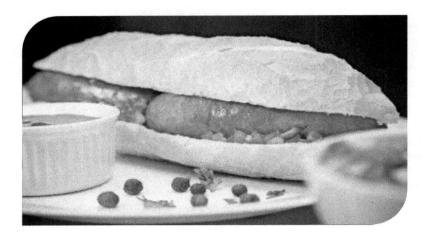

Ingredients

- 2 units of French bread
- 2 units of Tuscan sausage
- 3 ounces catupiry (3 tbsp)
- ½ unit of tomato without seeds cut

Steps to Cook

1. Remove sausage casing and larger fat.
2. Cut French bread in half lengthwise
3. Pass the catupiry on each bread
4. Spread over the catupiry cheese slices
5. Finish with the tomatoes.
6. Place in the deep fryer already heated to 390°F and leave for 10 minutes.

Nutrition Information

- Calories: 265
- Carbohydrates: 25.5g
- Fat: 13g
- Protein: 9g
- Sugar: 3g
- Cholesterol: 33mg

Australian Bread (Outback Style)

Servings: 4-6
Preparation time: 5 minutes
Cook time: 15 minutes

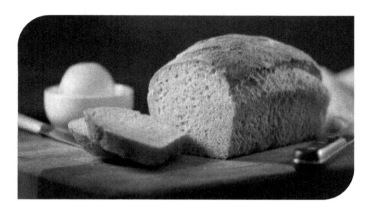

Ingredients

- 1 cup of water
- 1 tbsp butter
- 1 tbsp of oil
- ½ cup of honey
- 2 ½ cups white wheat flour
- 1 cup whole wheat flour
- 1 cup rye flour
- 2 tbsp cocoa powder (without sugar)
- 3 tbsp of brown sugar
- 1 tsp salt
- 2 ½ tsp dry organic yeast
- Corn flour for sprinkling

Steps to Cook

1. If you have a bread machine, add all the ingredients in the machine shape, starting with the liquids, then dry them, and finally the yeast and set the kneading or dough cycle, leave until the dough is well kneaded.
2. If you are going to do it by hand, put everything in a bowl and mix well until you get smooth and homogeneous dough.
3. Do not knead the dough on cold surfaces as it will affect growth.
4. Divide the dough into 6 equal parts and form baguettes, roll each baguette over the cornmeal, and then if you want to make cuts on top with a sharp cut.
5. Place on a baking sheet, cover with plastic wrap or put in a sachet and let it grow until it almost doubles its volume.
6. Preheat the Air Fryer for 5 minutes at 350°F, place two loaves of bread in the basket and program for 15 minutes at 350°F.
7. As soon as they are ready, carefully remove them and let them heat for at least 2 minutes before serving.
8. Serve warm or warm with butter.

Nutrition Information

- Calories: 191
- Carbohydrates: 30g
- Fat: 2g
- Protein: 9g
- Sugar: 1g
- Cholesterol: 300mg

Rustic potato

Servings: 4
Preparation time: 5 minutes
Cook time: 10 minutes

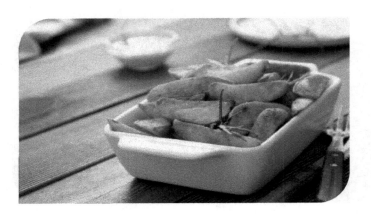

Ingredients

- 5 *large potatoes*
- 3 or 4 *branches of rosemary*
- 5 *garlic cloves*
- 3 *tbsp of coarse salt*

Steps to Cook

1. Wash the potatoes very well, removing all dirt from the skin.
2. Cook the potatoes with plenty of water, salt, and the rosemary sprigs with the loose leaves, until well cooked, but still firm.
3. Leave the potatoes in a colander until cool and refrigerate overnight.
4. After that time, cut the potatoes into 0.5 cm thick slices, keeping the skin on.
5. Reserve in the refrigerator until it is time to fry.
6. Heat the fryer at 350°F for 5 minutes, put a tablespoon of oil in a container. Add the potatoes and butter lightly. Place the potatoes in the fryer drawer and leave until golden brown, stirring occasionally. In the middle of the preparation, place the garlic cloves, so that they do not burn.
7. Decorate with rosemary, sprinkle with salt and serve.

Nutrition Information

- Calories: 291.5
- Carbohydrates: 66.7g
- Fat: 0.3g
- Protein: 7.9g
- Sugar: 2.3g
- Cholesterol: 45m

Onion Stuffed With Ricotta

Servings: 2
Preparation time: 5 minutes
Cook time: 10 minutes

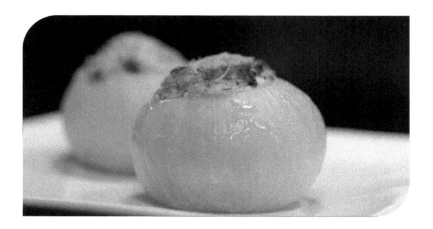

Ingredients

- 4 medium whole onions

Filling:

- 3 tbsp of extra virgin olive oil
- 1 ½ onion, diced into small cubes
- 1 cup half-moon leek
- 1 ripe peeled, ripe seedless tomato
- 1 tbsp chopped fresh basil
- 1 tbsp fresh marjoram
- 1 tbsp chopped chives
- 2 tbsp of breadcrumbs
- 2 cups crumbled ricotta
- 4 tbsp grated Parmesan cheese
- Salt and black pepper to taste.

To sprinkle:

Steps to Cook

1. Peel the onions and scoop out the kernels with a spoon, being careful not to pierce the bottom and side.
2. Bring a pot of water to a boil, put the onions in the water and boil for 10 minutes, remove from the boiling water, rinse with cold water to stop cooking, drain and set aside.
3. Chop the core of 2 onions into very small cubes and set aside.

For the filling:

1. Heat a frying pan well and add the oil, sauté the chopped onion and leeks until they wilt. Add diced tomatoes and cook until they start to crumble. Add the basil, marjoram, and breadcrumbs. Turn off the heat and allow the filling to cool slightly, and finally add the ricotta cheese, chives, and grated cheese.
1. Season the filling with salt and pepper.
2. Fill the precooked onions with the sautéed ricotta pressing well and sprinkle with Parmesan cheese grated on them.
3. Take the stuffed onions to roast in a preheated oven until the surface is golden brown.

- ½ cup grated Parmesan cheese

4. Preheated fryer at 390°F for 10 minutes.

Nutrition Information

- Calories: 265
- Carbohydrates: 25.5g
- Fat: 13g

- Protein: 9g
- Sugar: 3g
- Cholesterol: 33mg

Tomato Stuffed With Moroccan Couscous

Servings: 4
Preparation time: 30 minutes
Cook time: 15 minutes

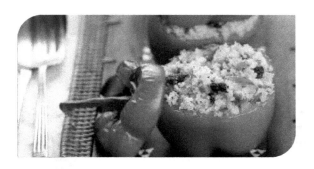

Ingredients

- 4 medium tomatoes

Filling:

- ½ cup chicken or vegetable broth
- ½ cup Moroccan couscous
- 1 tbsp butter
- 3 ½ oz. of salami
- 1 stalk of chopped leeks
- 1 medium grated carrot
- 1 tbsp finely chopped onion
- Tomato pulp (seedless)
- Olive oil
- Salt

Steps to Cook

1. In a frying pan prepare the broth and reserve.
2. Remove the lid from the tomatoes and reserve, with a spoon, remove the inside of the tomato, discard all the liquids and seeds and mince the pulp, pass a little salt inside the tomatoes and leave with the cut part to drain.
3. Finely chop the onion, place in a strainer, wash with warm water and set aside. In a frying pan place the finely chopped pepperoni with a drizzle of olive oil and sauté until golden, add the leek and brown, turn off the heat and add the grated carrot and the chopped tomato pulp and onion.
4. Preheat the air fryer at 350°F for a few minutes. Now heat the broth again, taste the salt, add half the butter, turn off the heat, add the couscous, cover the pan and let it hydrate for 5 minutes. After that time, mix the remaining butter, stir well so that the couscous is completely loose, and add the sautéed pepperoni and mix.
5. Place the tomatoes in a pan or ovenproof dish, fill the entire cavity with couscous, press lightly to fill well, put the tomato "lid" on and put in the air fryer for about 15 minutes.

Nutrition Information

- Calories: 235.1
- Carbohydrates: 45.1g
- Fat: 2.2g
- Protein: 9.14g
- Sugar: 0g
- Cholesterol: 3.6m

Delicious Garlic Bread

Servings: 4
Preparation time: 5 minutes
Cook time: 10 minutes

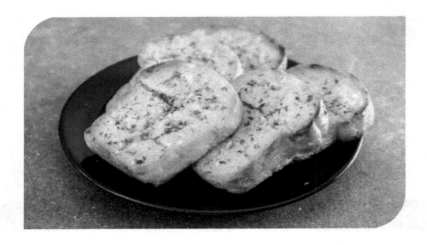

Ingredients

- 3 stale French rolls
- 4 tbsp minced or crushed garlic
- 1 cup butter or margarine
- Grated Parmesan cheese for sprinkling
- 1 tablespoon of olive oil

Steps to Cook

1. Preheat the air fryer to 390°F. Mix the butter or margarine with the garlic and set aside.
2. With the help of a brush, spread the oil over the rolls.
3. Cut the rolls into slices, but without separating them completely, and distribute the garlic paste in the cavities, evenly.
4. Close the rolls, sprinkle with the grated Parmesan cheese, and place them in the basket on the electric fryer.
5. Set the time for 10 minutes and set the temperature to 350°F.
6. At the end of time, your garlic breads will be ready to serve.

Nutrition Information

- Calories: 53
- Carbohydrates: 7.3g
- Fat: 2.04g
- Protein: 1.24g
- Sugar: 0.07g
- Cholesterol: 0mg

Crispy Vegetables

Servings: 2-4
Preparation time: 5 minutes
Cook time: 10 minutes

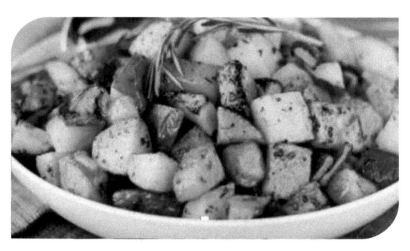

Ingredients

- 2 units of potato
- 1 unit of carrot
- salt to taste
- oregano to taste
- fine herbs to taste
- 3 tbsp of soybean oil

Steps to Cook

1. Cut the vegetables the way you prefer (chopsticks, slices, etc.). Brush the olive oil in the vegetables and season well, rubbing so that the seasoning passes through all the ingredients. Place in the fryer basket, and bake at 374°F for 10 minutes.
2. Remove the basket; stir the vegetables and place back to bake for another 10 minutes.
3. Keep dry and crispy. Bon appetite!

Nutrition Information

- Calories: 120
- Carbohydrates: 10.1g
- Fat: 8.3g
- Protein: 1.4g
- Sugar: 5.4g
- Cholesterol: 0mg

Rustic Sweet Potatoes Without Frying

Servings: 4-6
Preparation time: 10 mins
Cook time: 20 minutes

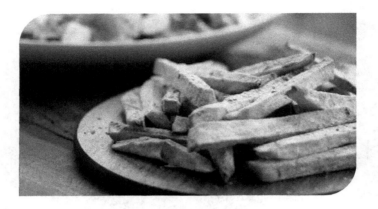

Ingredients

- 1 lb sweet potatoes
- 1 tbsp of wheat flour
- 1 garlic clove, finely chopped
- Herbs to taste (rosemary, fine herbs, oregano, thyme)
- ½ tbsp of olive oil
- Hot paprika (to taste)
- Salt

Steps to Cook

1. Heat the air fryer to 420°F.
2. Peel the potatoes and cut them into uniform sticks. Place the minced garlic clove, drizzle with olive oil and mix so that all the potatoes are lightly greased.
3. In a small bowl, mix together the flour, paprika and chosen herbs, mix and sprinkle the potatoes. Mix well so that the seasoned flour lightly touches all sides.
4. Place in the fryer or in a lightly greased pan to go to the oven and leave until the potatoes are soft on the inside and lightly browned on the outside. It took less than 20 minutes in the fryer.
5. Sprinkle with salt and pepper and serve.
6. Serve the potatoes with a salad of smashed lettuce leaves, sun-dried tomatoes, buffalo mozzarella, and walnuts.

Nutrition Information

- Calories: 291.5
- Carbohydrates: 66.7g
- Fat: 0.3g
- Protein: 7.9g
- Sugar: 2.3g
- Cholesterol: 45mg

Tuna And Sweet Potato

Servings: 2-4
Preparation time: 5 minutes
Cook time: 25 minutes

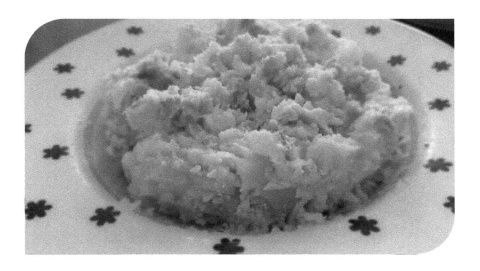

Ingredients

- 1 can of tuna
- 1 onion, chopped
- 1 tomato, chopped
- 2 tbsp of olive oil
- 1 cup chopped green
- 1 ½ cups sweet potatoes, boiled and mashed
- ½ cup milk
- 2 tbsp of margarine
- ½ jar of curd
- Salt and black pepper to taste.

Steps to Cook

1. Preheat the Air fryer to 390°F.
2. Place the drained tuna in a greased baking dish with oil and add the onion, green smell and chopped tomato. Add the black pepper. Place the refractory in the basket of the Air fryer and set the time to 5 minutes. Reserve.
3. Beat the sweet potato with the milk in a blender.
4. Add margarine and heat to thicken.
5. Put the salt. Remove from the heat and wait for it to heat up. Gently mix with the curd. Add over tuna in ovenproof dish. Return the refractory to the basket of the Air fryer and adjust the time to 20 minutes at 350°F. Serve!

Nutrition Information

- Calories: 120
- Carbohydrates: 10.1g
- Fat: 8.3g
- Protein: 1.4g
- Sugar: 5.4g
- Cholesterol: 0mg

Tapioca Dadinho

Servings: 2-4
Preparation time: 5 minutes
Cook time: 25 minutes

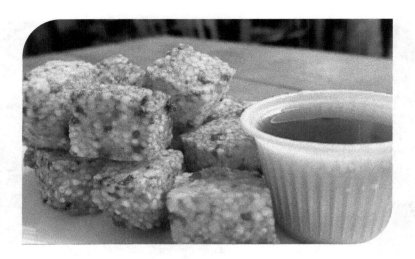

Ingredients

- 1 ½ cups tapioca, also known as tapioca flour
- 2 1/3 cups grated fresh rennet or Parmesan cheese
- 2 1/8 cup of very hot milk
- 1 teaspoon salt

Steps to Cook

1. Put the tapioca flour, cheese and salt in a bowl, mix and pour the hot milk on top, add another mixture and wait about 10 minutes for the flour to be absorbed by the tapioca flour, stirring occasionally. When. It will almost become soft dough.
2. Line a baking sheet with plastic and grease with oil and pour the mixture that you made on top, spread it out and place it with a spoon or spatula so that it is smooth and measures approximately 2.5 cm high.
3. Freeze for at least 3 hours.
4. With a knife cut into 2.5cm x 2.5cm cubes and set aside. Heat the Air Fryer for 5 minutes at 390°F, then place as many dice as you can in the Air Fryer's basket, without leaving one glued to the other, and set it for 15 minutes at 390°F and that's it. Ready!

Nutrition Information

- Calories: 92
- Carbohydrates: 6g
- Fat: 6g
- Protein: 2g
- Sugar: 0g
- Cholesterol: 300m

Australian Gluten Free Bread

Servings: 2-4
Preparation time: 5 minutes
Cook time: 1h 30 minutes

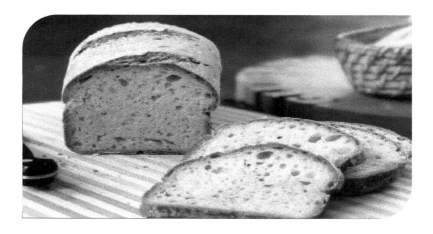

Ingredients

- 2 eggs
- 3 tbsp of honey
- 2 tbso of olive oil
- 1 tbsp of apple vinegar
- 1 tablet of fresh yeast
- ½ cup of rice flour
- ½ cup of precooked cornmeal
- 4 tbsp of powdered candy
- 4 tbsp of potato starch
- 3 tbsp of linseed flour
- 2 tbsp cocoa powder
- 4 tbsp of brown sugar
- ½ tbsp of salt

Steps to Cook

1. In a bowl, mix the eggs, honey, oil, vinegar, yeast, and ½ cup of warm water.
2. Stir well until the yeast dissolves.
3. Add the rest of the ingredients and mix until obtaining a homogeneous mass.
4. Pour the dough into an English cake pan (24 x 11 cm), greased with oil and sprinkled with Nestlé cocoa powder, and with the help of a spoon moistened with water, roll out and smooth the dough.
5. Cover with plastic wrap and let sit for 30 minutes.
6. With the help of a knife, make three cuts on the surface of the bread and sprinkle the cornmeal to finish.
7. Bake in the air fryer at 350°F, preheated, for approximately 40 minutes. Wait for it to cool, unmold and serve.

Nutrition Information

- Calories: 168
- Carbohydrates: 33g
- Fat: 1.4g
- Protein: 4.6g
- Sugar: 2.30g
- Cholesterol: 0mg

Damper

Servings: 2-4
Preparation time: 5 minutes
Cook time: 25 minutes

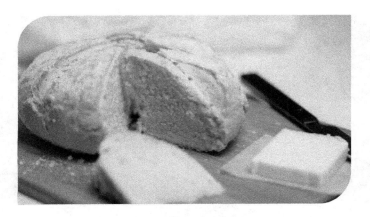

Ingredients

- 3 cups of wheat flour with yeast
- 1 ½ tbsp of salt
- 3 oz. of butter
- ½ cup milk
- ½ cup of water
- Extra flour

Steps to Cook

1. Sift the flour and salt into the pan, gently mix the butter with your fingers and mix until it forms homogeneous dough. Or even mix in the processor. Make a circle in the center of the dry ingredients, add the water mixed with the milk, all at once, mix lightly with a sharp knife making cutting movements.
2. Remove only the surface of the flour, knead lightly.
3. Roll the dough into a round shape until it is 18 cm in diameter. Knead the dough in circles and place it in the form of brushed butter. Using a sharp knife, make two narrow, cross-shaped cuts about 2 cm deep.
4. Sprinkle the top of the dough with milk; sprinkle a little more flour on the dough.
5. Put in the air fryer for 10 minutes at $390°F$.
6. Reduce the temperature to moderate and bake for another 15 minutes.

Nutrition Information

- Calories: 168
- Carbohydrates: 33g
- Fat: 1.4g
- Protein: 4.6g
- Sugar: 2.30g
- Cholesterol: 0mg

Leaf Bread

Servings: 2-4
Preparation time: 5 minutes
Cook time: 25 minutes

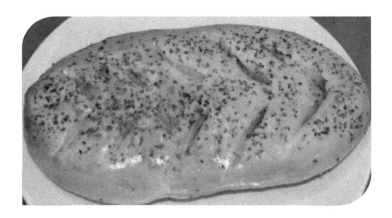

Ingredients

- 1 ½ cup whole wheat flour
- 1 ½ cup of white wheat flour
- ½ tsp salt
- ¾ cup warm water
- 3 tbsp butter or margarine
- ½ tbsp (brown) of dry or fresh yeast

Steps to Cook

1. In a bowl put all the ingredients and mix well, until obtaining a smooth and homogeneous mass.
2. If you have a bread machine, you can prepare it using the pasta cycle. As soon as the dough is done, roll into a ball and brush with a few drops of olive oil, then cover with a plastic wrap or put it in a sachet and let it sit for 30 minutes. After the dough rest time, divide the dough ball into 12 balls.
3. Preheat the Air Fryer and in the meantime start rolling the balls open, opening it very thin, like very thin pancake dough, in a circular shape, about the size of the Air Fryer's basket more or less.
4. Place a loaf of bread in the Air Fryer basket and program for 3 minutes at 390°F. When it is done, the bread will be slightly golden and puffy.

Nutrition Information

- Calories: 168
- Carbohydrates: 33g
- Fat: 1.4g
- Protein: 4.6g
- Sugar: 2.30g
- Cholesterol: 0mg

French Cheese Fries

Servings: 4-6
Preparation time: 5 minutes
Cook time: 25 minutes

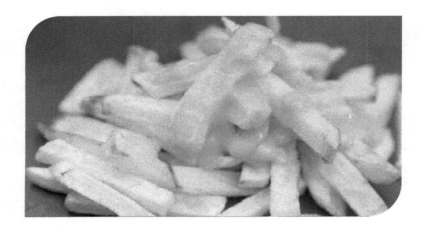

Ingredients

- 1 lb of potatoes cut into thin strips
- 4 slices of chopped cheddar cheese
- 3 tbsp of curd
- 1 pinch of black pepper
- 4 slices of bacon

Steps to Cook

1. Preheat the air fryer at 390°F for a few minutes. Then, put the potatoes for 20 minutes.
2. Remove and set aside.
3. Melt the curd and the minced cheddar cheese and mix a lot (it will form a very orange cream), add the black pepper and reserve.
4. Wrap the bacon slices in paper towels and put in the air fryer at 150°C for 4 minutes.
5. It will be super crispy and dry.
6. Break the slices and reserve.
7. Arrange the potatoes on a plate, spread the cheese sauce on top gently and sprinkle on the crispy bacon.

Nutrition Information

- Calories: 280
- Carbohydrates: 29g
- Fat: 15g
- Protein: 6g
- Sugar: 1g
- Cholesterol: 20mg

Pizza With Homemade Dough

Servings: 4-6
Preparation time: 10 minutes
Cook time: 8 minutes

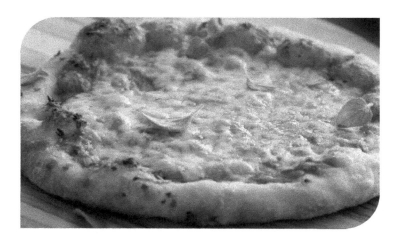

Ingredients

- 1 cup warm milk with 1 egg inside
- 1/3 cup warm water
- ¼ cup of olive oil
- 2 tbsp of salt
- 2 tbsp of sugar
- 2 ½ tsp of dry yeast or 2 tablets of fresh yeast
- 4 cups of flour
- Ingredients of your choice: tomato sauce, olives, olive oil and oregano.

Steps to Cook

1. Mix all the ingredients in a bowl and knead well until you get smooth and homogeneous dough.
2. Be careful not to add too much flour and make the dough hard or heavy.
3. Once the dough is ready, separate it into 10 equal parts, roll it into balls and open it with a circular disk-shaped roller, they should be almost the size of the Air Fryer basket. Once this is done, place one disc at a time in the Air Fryer basket, already preheated, and program for 3 minutes at 390°F.
4. Remove from the basket and repeat the process with the remaining pasta discs.
5. To prepare the pizza put a little sauce on the dough disk and spread it out well, put the desired coverage, add olives, sprinkle oregano and olive oil to taste.
6. Place the pizza in the Air Fryer basket and place it for 5 minutes at 390°F and ready.

Nutrition Information

- Calories: 72
- Carbohydrates: 13g
- Fat: 1.3g
- Protein: 1.8g
- Sugar: 0.6g
- Cholesterol: 0mg

Bread With Egg

Servings: 2-4
Preparation time: 5 minutes
Cook time: 8 minutes

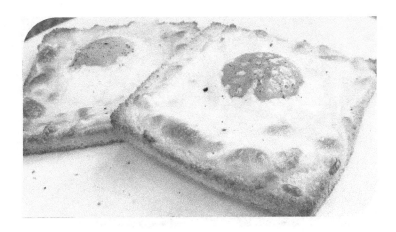

Ingredients

Pasta:
- 1 cup warm milk with 1 egg inside (put the egg in the cup and then fill it with milk)
- 1/3 cup warm water
- ¼ cup oil or olive oil
- 2 tsp of salt
- 2 tbsp of sugar
- 2 ½ tsp of dry yeast
- 4 cups of wheat flour

Filling:
- 10 eggs

Steps to Cook

1. Mix all the ingredients in a bowl and knead well until you get smooth and homogeneous dough.
2. Be careful not to add too much flour and make the dough hard or heavy. If you have a bread machine, just put everything inside the machine shape and set the kneading or dough cycle for at least 30 minutes, then remove and use the dough.
3. As soon as the dough is ready, separate it into 10 equal parts, form each piece of dough as if it were a small pot, a crumb, and then put the egg inside and bake everything together.
4. Place two molded doughs inside the Air Fryer basket, break one egg into each and sprinkle a little salt on top. Program the Air Fryer for 8 minutes at 390°F.

Nutrition Information

- Calories: 166.6
- Carbohydrates: 19.5g
- Fat: 2.4g
- Protein: 3.9g
- Sugar: 0.7g
- Cholesterol: 20.7mg

Australian Panettone

Servings: 2-4
Preparation time: 5 minutes
Cook time: 8 minutes

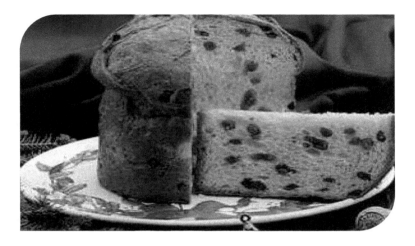

Ingredients

- 1 tbsp of baking powder
- 7 mashed dwarf bananas
- ½ cup of ground walnuts
- 2 ½ cup breadcrumbs
- 2 cups of sugar
- 1 cup of oil
- 3 egg whites
- 3 gems

Steps to Cook

1. Beat the egg whites.
2. Beat the egg yolks with the sugar until white; add the oil, the banana and nuts mixed with the breadcrumbs, the yeast and finally the egg whites.
3. Take to air fryer at 390°F for only 8 minutes in the form of sweet bread.
4. Stick a toothpick to see if it is roasted.
5. Take it out of the air fryer and cover it, while the cake is hot with lemon and icing sugar and spread it over the ground walnut.
6. If you want you can add a tablespoon of vanilla essence.

Nutrition Information

- Calories: 326
- Carbohydrates: 63g
- Fat: 6.4g
- Protein: 6.4g
- Sugar: 29g
- Cholesterol: 51mg

Puff Pastry

Servings: 2-4
Preparation time: 5 minutes
Cook time: 10 minutes

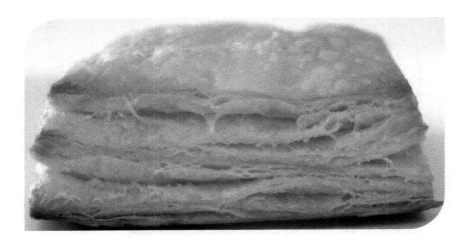

Ingredients

- Yolk
- Grated cheese
- crystal sugar, seeds or grains

Steps to Cook

1. Cut the puff pastry into small, thin strips, and then brush with egg yolk on top, sprinkle the coverage you chose on top.
2. Now take each strip of puff pastry and twist it, then place it in the Air Fryer basket.
3. Adjust the Air Fryer for 10 minutes at 390°F. Serve as soon as the time is up.
4. You can sprinkle with sugars, sprinkled sweets or grated cheeses, seeds like sesame, chia, flaxseed, you can also sprinkle with dry tomato oil or anchovies, and they will be beautiful and tasty!

Nutrition Information

- Calories: 158
- Carbohydrates: 13g
- Fat: 11g
- Protein: 2.1g
- Sugar: 0.2g
- Cholesterol: 0mg

Fried Egg

Servings: 1
Preparation time: 5 minutes
Cook time: 10 minutes

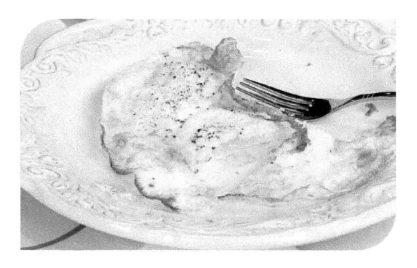

Ingredients

- 1 egg

Steps to Cook

1. Separate a porcelain or glass plate, it can also be a dessert plate, but it has a deeper center and higher edges, and of course it has to fit inside the Air Fryer basket.
2. Grease the dish with oil, cooking oil, butter or margarine, place it in the preheated Air Fryer basket and gently break the egg in the center.
3. Sprinkle salt on top.
4. Adjust the Air Fryer to 390°F for the 5 minutes.

Nutrition Information

- Calories: 90
- Carbohydrates: 0.6g
- Fat: 7g
- Protein: 6.3g
- Sugar: 0g
- Cholesterol: 210mg

Mexican Lentils

Servings: 2-4
Preparation time: 5 minutes
Cook time: 10 minutes

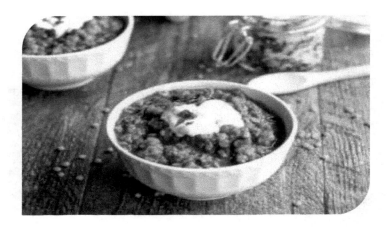

Ingredients

- 1 lb lentils
- ½ lb of bacon
- Fat-free chicken broth
- 3 garlic cloves
- 4 tomatoes
- ½ onion
- Parsley

Steps to Cook

1. Wash the lentils well, boil in 4 cups of water.
2. Chop the bacon into cubes and put in the air fryer at 390°F for 10 minutes.
3. Remove this fat and leave a little to skip the sauce.
4. In a blender, grind tomatoes, onions, garlic, and a little water.
5. Skip this sauce. Add the chopped parsley and fried bacon and season with the chicken stock.
6. When the lentil is almost cooked, add this sauce.
7. If needed more salt, add until you like it.
8. When serving, you can squeeze a lemon into the soup.

Nutrition Information

- Calories: 90
- Carbohydrates: 0.6g
- Fat: 7g

- Protein: 6.3g
- Sugar: 0g
- Cholesterol: 210mg

Chapter 3

Air Fryer Snacks and Appetizers

Anzac Cookie

Servings: 4-6
Preparation time: 5 minutes
Cook time: 15-20 minutes

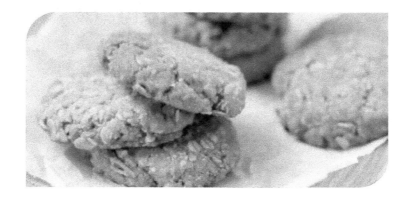

Ingredients

- 3 ½ oz. rolled oats
- 5 oz. wheat flour, sifted
- 7 oz. of refined sugar
- 2 ½ oz. of grated coconut
- 4 ½ oz. of butter
- 2 tbsp of molasses
- 1 ½ tbsp baking soda, sifted

Steps to Cook

1. Smash all dry ingredients except the baking soda.
2. In a small saucepan, heat butter and molasses and mix until melted. Mix the baking soda and mix well.
3. Place in the center of the dry ingredients and mix well with a spoon. Place the cookies in molds lined with non-stick paper, with approximately 5 cm of space between them.
4. Put in the air fryer at 350°F for 15 to 20 minutes, until golden.
5. Serve immediately.

Nutrition Information

- Calories: 123
- Carbohydrates: 16g
- Fat: 5g
- Protein: 1g
- Sugar: 9g
- Cholesterol: 300mg

Apple Pie Australian

Servings: 4
Preparation time: 15 minutes
Cook time: 40 minutes

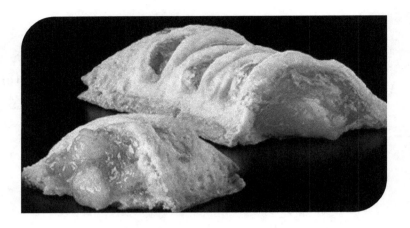

Ingredients

- 1 Australian wick bread
- 6 Argentine apples
- 4 tsp of butter
- 1 cup of tea
- Juice of 2 oranges
- 3 spoonfuls of sugar
- 2 butter spoons

Steps to Cook

1. Grease four baking pans (22 cm X 6 cm) with butter and sprinkle the bottom of each with 3 tablespoons of sugar.
2. On a cutting board, cut the apples in half and remove the brains (part where the seeds are). Then place them center down. Use a knife to cut them into thin strips, fan-shaped, as in the photo above.
3. Remove the ends of the bread with a thickness of two fingers. Cut the rest into four equal parts, lengthwise.
4. Chop the ends and set aside. Place three apple halves on each baking sheet, skin side down.
5. Top with a long slice of bread and drizzle each with a little orange juice.
6. Put in the preheated air fryer at 350°F for 40 minutes, or until the bread is crisp and the apples are soft.

Nutrition Information

- Calories: 61
- Carbohydrates: 13g
- Fat: 0g
- Protein: 0g
- Sugar: 13g
- Cholesterol: 300mg

Greek Barbecue/Kebab

Servings: 2-3
Preparation time: 10 minutes
Cook time: 35 minutes

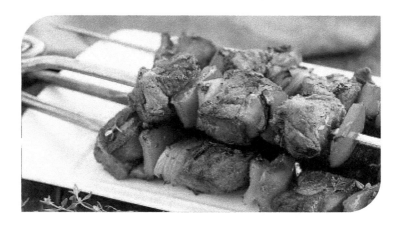

Ingredients

- 1 ½ lb of meat in fillets, can be meatloaf, fillet, loin, limp or duckling, it can even be a mixture of several of these.
- ½ green bell pepper, finely sliced
- ½ red or yellow bell pepper, finely sliced
- 1 small onion
- Salt and black pepper

Steps to Cook

1. Remove the basket from the Air Fryer and place it on a flat surface, place a fillet in the center of the basket and place a little of each pepper, onion, salt and pepper on top, place another fillet on top and repeat the process making several layers and finish with meat.
2. Now cover these meats with a piece of aluminum foil, place the basket, and place them in the Air Fryer. Program for 25 minutes at 350°F.
3. After this time, open the Air Fryer, remove the foil from the meat and place it for another 10 minutes at 200°C. Remove from Air Fryer and place it on a cutting board, cut the meat finely with a sharp knife, place it on a French roll and serve.

Nutrition Information

- Calories: 145
- Carbohydrates: 1g
- Fat: 5g
- Protein: 21g
- Sugar: 0g
- Cholesterol: 300mg

Roasted Peanuts

Servings: 12
Preparation time: 1 minute
Cook time: 35 minutes

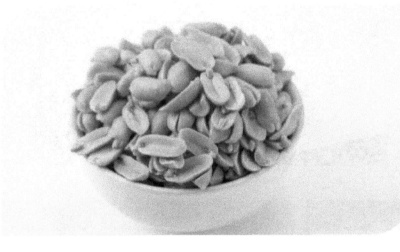

Ingredients

- 1 lb raw peanuts
- 2 tbsp of oil
- 2 tbsp of water
- 1 tbsp of salt

Steps to Cook

1. For shelled/skinless peanuts, place them in a bowl and pour oil, water, and salt over them, mix well, and place them in the Air Fryer basket.
2. Adjust the Air Fryer for 20 minutes at 360°F, remembering to shake the basket every 5 minutes so that the peanuts are toasted evenly.
3. Then remove and pour into a bowl, let it heat up or cool down and rub the peanuts with your hands, it can even blow, the shells will come out easily.
4. After peeling and discarding the shells, add oil, water, and salt.
5. Adjust the Air Fryer for 15 minutes at 390°F, shaking the basket every 5 minutes to toast it evenly.

Nutrition Information

- Calories: 165
- Carbohydrates: 5.5g
- Fat: 14g
- Protein: 7g
- Sugar: 2g
- Cholesterol: 0mg

Banana Chips

Servings: 1-2
Preparation time: 5 minutes
Cook time: 20-25 minutes

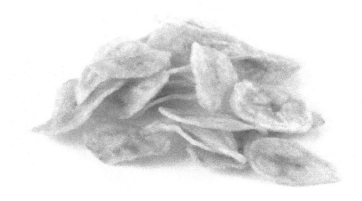

Ingredients

- *Green bananas*
- *Salt or sugar to taste*

Steps to Cook

1. Peel the banana, then cut it with a sharp 2 mm (0.2 cm) thick knife, no need to rush, green banana does not brown as fast as the ripe one.
2. Put the slices in the Air Fryer basket carefully and sprinkle a little salt or sugar, depending on whether you want sweet or salty chips, if you want you can also do it with nothing, it will work the same way.
3. Adjust the Air Fryer for 20 to 25 minutes at 300°F, until they are dry and lightly browned, then remove them from the basket and add another batch.
4. After removing the banana chips from the Air Fryer, let them cool down so you can store them in a tightly closed jar or bag.

Nutrition Information

- Calories: 114
- Carbohydrates: 13g
- Fat: 5.9g
- Protein: 2.3g
- Sugar: 3.2g
- Cholesterol: 19mg

Fugazza

Servings: 7
Preparation time: 20 minutes
Cook time: 8 minutes

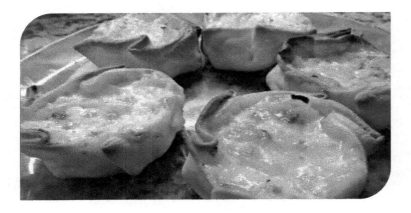

Ingredients

- 1 cup warm milk
- 3 tbsp olive oil
- 2 tbsp of sugar
- 1 tbsp of salt
- 3 cups of flour
- 3 tbsp of yeast

Filling:

- ½ lb of mozzarella grated, crushed or finely chopped
- ½ cup seedless tomatoes, diced
- 1 tbsp of fresh basil

Steps to Cook

1. Mix all the ingredients of the dough and knead until you get a smooth and uniform dough, then place in a bowl and cover with a cloth or plastic and let stand for 20 minutes. After the rest of the dough has passed, grease a smooth surface with oil or olive oil and place the dough, divide it into 7 parts and make a ball with each part of the dough.
2. Take a ball of dough and flatten it and press it on the surface with olive oil, it will open easily, without the need for a roll, only in the hand.
3. Put the filling, fold it in half and close the edges, pressing with a fork to both sides of the fire so that it does not open when frying.
4. Put two hot puffs in the Air Fryer basket at the same time, adjust for 8 minutes at 400°F, when the time is up, remove the hot pans from the Air Fryer and repeat the process with the rest until the end.

Nutrition Information

- Calories: 210
- Carbohydrates: 29g
- Fat: 8g
- Protein: 5g
- Sugar: 1g
- Cholesterol: 300mg

Antipasto

Servings: 2-4
Preparation time: 5 minutes
Cook time: 30 minutes

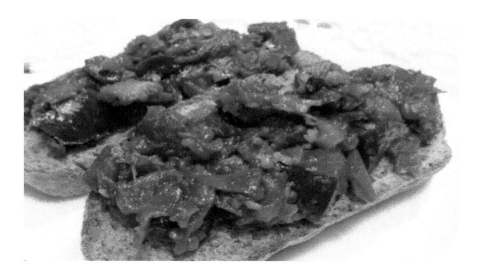

Ingredients

- 1 aubergine
- ½ green pepper
- ½ red pepper
- ½ yellow pepper
- 1 medium onion
- ½ cup (olives)
- 1 head of garlic
- 3 tbsp olive oil
- ½ tsp salt
- Black pepper to taste
- 2 tbsp of vinegar
- Olive oil to taste

Steps to Cook

1. Cut the eggplant into cubes and the peppers and onion into slices of approximately 0.5 cm.
2. Peel the garlic and cut it into thin slices.
3. Put everything in a bowl and add the olive oil, olives, salt and pepper. Mix everything well and put it in the Air Fryer basket, it will be very full.
4. Program the Air Fryer for 10 minutes at 180°C.
5. At the end of this time, stir to rotate and cook evenly.
6. Now program the Air Fryer for 20 minutes at 400°F, always stirring every 7 minutes or so.
7. Once ready, place it in a bowl and add vinegar and more oil to taste.

Nutrition Information

- Calories: 240
- Carbohydrates: 9g
- Fat: 13g
- Protein: 22g
- Sugar: 6g
- Cholesterol: 70mg

Mozzarella Sticks

Servings: 2-4
Preparation time: 2 minutes
Cook time: 7 minutes

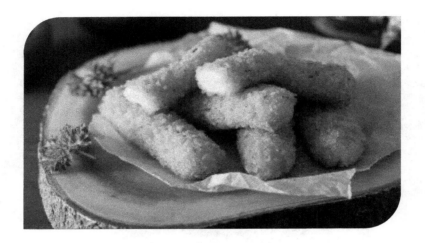

Ingredients

- ½ lb of mozzarella
- 4 eggs
- 2 cups of wheat flour
- 2 cups of panko flour
- ½ tsp salt
- ½ tsp of oregano
- 1 pinch of black pepper

Steps to Cook

1. Cut the mozzarella into strips of 1 cm x 1 cm and use.
2. Place the eggs in a bowl and together with them the salt, oregano and black pepper, beat lightly and reserve.
3. Put the wheat flour in one bowl and the panko floor in another.
4. Now bread each stick of cheese passing first the eggs, then the wheat flour, again the eggs and again the wheat flour, finally the eggs and finally the panko flour.
5. Carry out the process with all the cheese sticks, being careful not to leave holes in the breading or excess flour.
6. Place the chopsticks on a baking sheet and place them in the freezer or freezer for at least 4 hours.
7. Once frozen, the sticks can now be prepared in the Air Fryer.
8. Place a maximum of half the recipe in the Air Fryer basket, alternating horizontally and vertically, then

program the Air Fryer for 7 minutes at 400°F.
9. They will only be slightly browned, but crispy and dry on the outside and the mozzarella melted on the inside.

Nutrition Information

- Calories: 100.8
- Carbohydrates: 7.8g
- Fat: 5.7g

- Protein: 4.6g
- Sugar: 0.7g
- Cholesterol: 11.2mg

Portuguese Chestnut

Servings: 4
Preparation time: 2 minutes
Cook time: 25 minutes

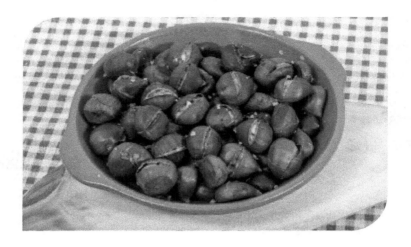

Ingredients

- ½ lb of Portuguese chestnuts
- 1 tbso butter
- 1 tsp of shallow salt

Steps to Cook

1. Wash the chestnuts well to remove dirt, then make cuts right in the middle, in the most rounded part, with a knife, cutting the peel until it reaches the chestnut, and give it a bit on the chestnut, a blow to make it loosen and then open more easily.
2. Place the chestnuts in the Air Fryer basket and pour the melted butter on them, then sprinkle the salt, stir and adjust the Air Fryer for 25 minutes at 400°F, shaking the basket approximately half the time so that it is uniform.
5. At the end, pour the chestnuts into a bowl and enjoy.

Nutrition Information

- Calories: 333
- Carbohydrates: 78.85g
- Fat: 2.44g
- Protein: 4.51g
- Sugar: 9.65g
- Cholesterol: 0mg

Cassava Dumpling With Dried Meat Filling

Servings: 40
Preparation time: 20 minutes
Cook time: 7 minutes

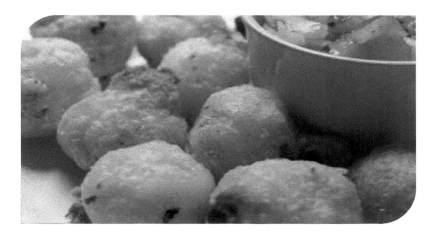

Ingredients

Mass:
- 2 ½ lb cassava cooked in salted water
- 2 gems
- ½ tbsp unsalted butter
- 1 tbsp of salt
- 2 tbsp of chopped parsley
- Black pepper to taste
- Wheat flour

Stuffed with dried meat:
- 1 tbsp olive oil
- 1 clove garlic, minced
- ½ chopped onion
- ½ lb desalinated and minced meat

To bread:
- 1 cup breadcrumbs
- 2 eggs

Steps to Cook

1. Preheat the Air fryer to 400°F for 3 minutes. Drain the cassava cooking water completely. Knead while it is still hot with a fork. Let it cool down.
2. In a bowl, mix all the ingredients of the dough well until it forms smooth dough, if necessary add wheat flour until it begins to come out of the hand. Reserve.

Filling:

3. In a skillet, add the oil and sauté the onion and garlic until lightly browned. Add the grated dried meat and sauté for a few more minutes.
4. To assemble, place ½ tbsp of the cassava dough in the palm of your hand, open a disk of the dough and place a spoon of filling. Close the disc over the filling and mold with both hands until it forms a cookie.
5. To beat, in a bowl, beat the eggs well and, in another, put the breadcrumbs. Roll the dumplings first over the eggs and then over the flour.
6. Transfer cookies to the Air fryer.
7. Fry them for 15 minutes, stirring every 4 minutes to brown them evenly.

Nutrition Information

- Calories: 348
- Carbohydrates: 24.61g
- Fat: 22.14g
- Protein: 12.16g
- Sugar: 0.13g
- Cholesterol: 23mg

Kibbeh Fried

Servings: 20
Preparation time: 30 minutes
Cook time: 18 minutes

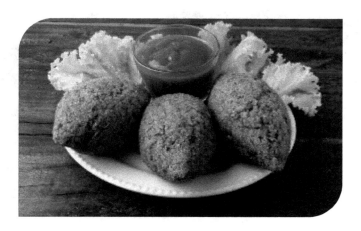

Ingredients

- 1 lb of wheat for kibbeh
- 1 kg ground duckling
- Condiments: salt, black pepper, mint, garlic, basil, parsley, turmeric
- 1 pinch ground cinnamon
- 4 cups of boiling water
- 4 tbsp of olive oil
- 2 tbsp of vinegar
- 3 ½ oz. pitted green olives

Steps to Cook

1. Boil a liter of water and place on the wheat.
2. Use a large bowl as the wheat doubles in volume.
3. Cover this bowl and let the mixture sit for 30 minutes.
4. In a processor, mix together all the spices, vinegar, cinnamon, olives and two tablespoons of oil.
5. Season the meat with this processed seasoning.
6. Take ¼ of the wheat and beat in the processor until you release an alloy. Mix all the ingredients. Put the salt. Shape the kibbeh. Before "frying" in the Air fryer, grease them with the rest of the oil.
7. Heat the Air fryer for 3 minutes at 400^0F.
8. Bake at 350^0F for 15 minutes, rotating the kibbeh for half that time.

Nutrition Information

- Calories: 160
- Carbohydrates: 6g
- Fat: 12g
- Protein: 9g
- Sugar: 0g
- Cholesterol: 265mg

Rain Balls

Servings: 2-4
Preparation time: 5 minutes
Cook time: 10 minutes

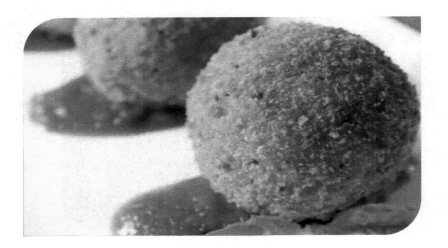

Ingredients

- 1 cup milk
- ½ cup of sugar
- 1 pinch of salt
- 2 tbsp melted margarine
- 2 ½ cups of wheat flour
- 1 tbsp baking powder

Coverage:

- 1 cup of sugar
- 1 tbsp ground cinnamon

Steps to Cook

1. In a bowl, mix all the ingredients and stir until it becomes a homogeneous dough
2. Meanwhile, allow the fryer to preheat to 400°F for 5 minutes. Then, with two spoons, form a little of the dough, creating a ball
3. Place the balls in the basket of the air fryer, leaving a space for your fingers between them so that they do not stick, and adjust the machine to 400°F for 6 minutes. The cookies will have a golden surface, remove them carefully and reserve!

Coverage:

4. Mix sugar and cinnamon powder.
5. Make all the cookies, roll them into the mix.

Nutrition Information

- Calories: 15
- Carbohydrates: 3g
- Fat: 1.5g
- Protein: 1g
- Sugar: 3g
- Cholesterol: 300mg

Rolls Ham And Cheese

Servings: 2
Preparation time: 5 minutes
Cook time: 7 minutes

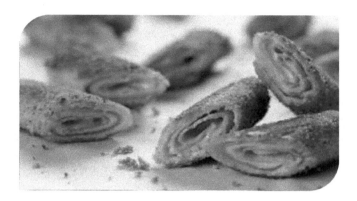

Ingredients

- Precooked lasagna dough, or puff pastry
- Sliced mozzarella cheese
- Sliced ham or turkey breast
- Tomato sauce or tomato sauce
- Mayonnaise
- Oregano

Steps to Cook

1. In rectangular dough, either lasagna or cake, place a tablespoon of tomato sauce or tomato sauce.
2. Then add 1 slice of mozzarella and 1 slice of ham or turkey breast
3. Add 1 tablespoon of mayonnaise and spread
4. Carefully close the roll, like a cake
5. Using a fork, press down on the sides to close it firmly
6. To leave a golden cone, place 1 extra tablespoon of mayonnaise on top, spreading over the entire surface
7. Put the rolls in your air fryer basket for 7 minutes at 350^0F.
8. Then sprinkle some oregano and serve.

Nutrition Information

- Calories: 267
- Carbohydrates: 20g
- Fat: 16g
- Protein: 12g
- Sugar: 1.6g
- Cholesterol: 61mg

Rice Balls

Servings: 2-4
Preparation time: 5 minutes
Cook time: 20 minutes

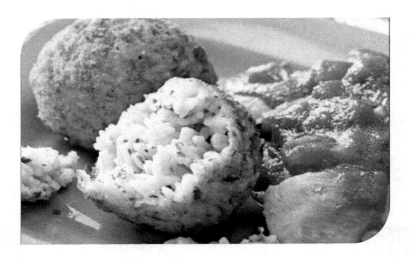

Ingredients

- 2 cups of cooked rice
- 1 cup grated cheese
- 2 eggs
- 1 cup all-purpose flour

Spices to taste:

- black pepper, oregano, chives, parsley and salt, if necessary

Steps to Cook

1. Mix all the ingredients and make balls.
2. Take to the fryer for 15 to 20 minutes at 350°F.

Nutrition Information

- Calories: 47
- Carbohydrates: 5.4g
- Fat: 2g
- Protein: 1.7g
- Sugar: 0.2g
- Cholesterol: 9.7mg

Patty

Servings: 2-4
Preparation time: 5 minutes
Cook time: 10 minutes

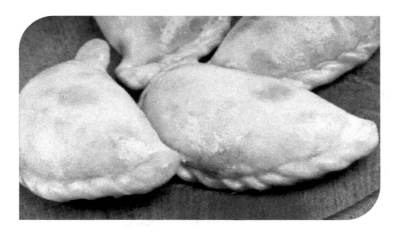

Ingredients

- *Fresh pastry for prepared pastry*
- *Stuffed to taste*

suggestions:

- *ground beef, shredded chicken, cheese, shitake, hearts of palm*

Steps to Cook

1. Open the dough and place the filling.
2. Close the dough with the tip of the fork.
3. Brush the dough with olive oil so it doesn't dry out.
4. Then place in the 350°F preheated fryer and leave for 10 minutes
5. The time may vary according to your preference. If you like the lighter dough, leave less time; if you prefer more gold, leave more

Nutrition Information

- Calories: 197
- Carbohydrates: 10g
- Fat: 12g
- Protein: 21g
- Sugar: 0g
- Cholesterol: 0mg

Bolovo

Servings: 6-10
Preparation time: 7 minutes
Cook time: 15 minutes

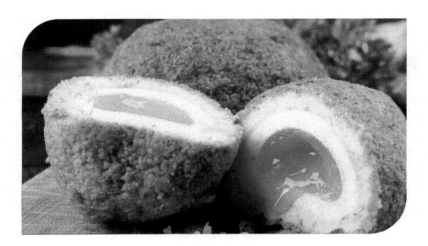

Ingredients

- 6 eggs
- 1 lb of ground meat
- 2 garlic cloves, crushed
- 1 tbsp of mustard (optional)
- salt to taste
- black pepper to taste

Steps to Cook

1. Cook 5 eggs for 7 minutes (the other egg goes in the dough)
2. Season the meat with garlic, mustard, salt and pepper, add the raw egg
3. Mix everything very well
4. Divide the meat into 5 servings of 3 ½ oz. each
5. Peel the eggs and wrap them with the meat, completely covering the egg.
6. Bake in the air fryer for 15 minutes at 400°F

Nutrition Information

- Calories: 235
- Carbohydrates: 10.34g
- Fat: 10.98g
- Protein: 23.19g
- Sugar: 1.1g
- Cholesterol: 66mg

Conservation Of Cod In Italian Bread

Servings: 4
Preparation time: 5 minutes
Cook time: 10 minutes

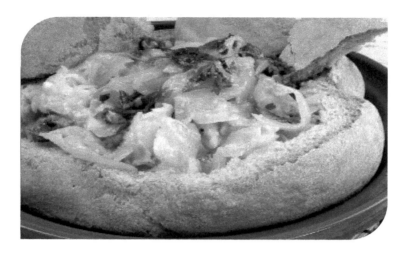

Ingredients

- ½ lb cod desalted in pieces
- 1 red bell pepper cut into squares
- 1 onion cut into petals
- 3 garlic cloves, thinly sliced
- 1 tbsp of capers
- 1 tbsp of pepper dessert
- Salt and pepper
- 1 Italian bread without crumbs, greased with oil and rubbed with ½ garlic clove

Steps to Cook

1. Prepare the cod and place it in a bowl.
2. Fry the garlic cloves in a little oil, then the onion and finally the pepper. Drain well and add to the cod.
3. Mix the remaining spices. Correct the salt and add black pepper. Place in a suitable container to keep it properly sterilized and add the oil.
4. Marinate for at least 4 days.
5. To serve, scoop out grains from skillet, keep lid, remove excess beans and rub with ½ clove garlic, moisten with olive oil.
6. Put in the air fryer for 10 minutes at 320°F for crisp without toasting too much. Add canned oil and cover.
7. Leave 5 minutes and serve.

Nutrition Information

- Calories: 216.8
- Carbohydrates: 5.9g
- Fat: 6.7g
- Protein: 31.5g
- Sugar: 0.7g
- Cholesterol: 133.4mg

Crutones

Servings: 2-3
Preparation time: 5 minutes
Cook time: 5 minutes

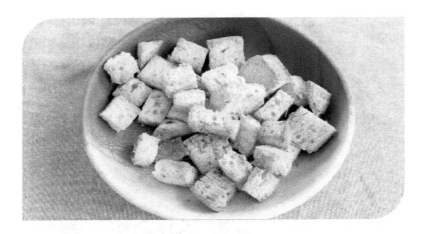

Ingredients

- *Bread cut into cubes.*
- *enough olive oil*
- *Dried oregano*
- *salt and pepper to taste*

Steps to Cook

1. Mix the bread, olive oil to taste, oregano, salt and pepper.
2. Heat the Air fryer for 5 minutes at 390°F.
3. Put it in the basket and with 30 seconds look to see if it is toasted and crispy. If it isn't already, add another 30 seconds until it turns into a crunchy crumb.

Nutrition Information

- Calories: 66
- Carbohydrates: 9g
- Fat: 0.8g
- Protein: 1.5g
- Sugar: 0.6g
- Cholesterol: 1mg

Tomato And Cheese Bruschetta

Servings: 2-4
Preparation time: 5 minutes
Cook time: 15 minutes

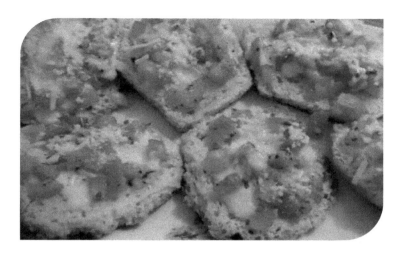

Ingredients

- 1 small Italian bread (or bread of your choice)
- 1 tomato
- 1 ½ oz. of mozzarella cheese
- 1 ½ oz. of grated parmesan cheese
- 1 clove garlic
- Olive oil to taste
- Dried basil to taste
- Salt and pepper to taste
- 1 tbsp butter

Steps to Cook

1. Start by cutting the tomatoes into slices. Take the seeds and cut them into small cubes.
2. Cut the mozzarella into small cubes as well. If you prefer, instead of mozzarella, you can add the cheese of your choice. Mix the two in a bowl and add salt, pepper, and basil (if you have fresh basil, the better). Drizzle with plenty of olive oil. Finely chop the garlic and mix.
3. Cut the loaves, pass a little butter and put in a pan. Put the mixture on top and add a little grated Parmesan cheese.
4. Place in a preheated air fryer at 390°F for about 15 minutes.

Nutrition Information

- Calories: 277.3
- Carbohydrates: 30.2g
- Fat: 10.4g
- Protein: 14.2g
- Sugar: 1g
- Cholesterol: 21.4mg

American Rosca Recipe

Servings: 20
Preparation time: 1 minute
Cook time: 35 minutes

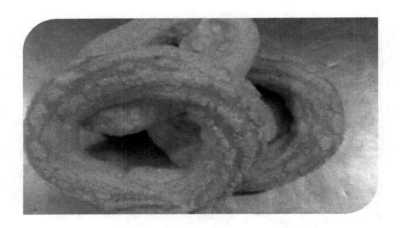

Ingredients

- 2 cups of milk
- 2 cups of oil
- 5 eggs
- 3 ½ oz. of sugar
- 2 ¼ lbs of powdered sugar

Steps to Cook

1. Put all the ingredients in a bowl. Mix everything with a large spoon, until well mixed without lumps. Then put it in a pastry bag with a large pitanga beak. Rectangular shaped model oiled with margarine. Make the donuts, put crystal sugar on top. Put in the air fryer at 302°F for 20 minutes.

Nutrition Information

- Calories: 290
- Carbohydrates: 36g
- Fat: 15g
- Protein: 4g
- Sugar: 8g
- Cholesterol: 0mg

Granola Cookies

Servings: 1-2
Preparation time: 5 minutes
Cook time: 8 minutes

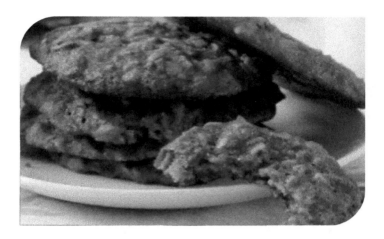

Ingredients

- 2 cups brown sugar
- 2 cups of almond flour or another of your choice
- Cinnamon to taste
- 2 eggs
- 1 cup granola
- 1 tbsp baking powder

Steps to Cook

1. Put everything in a large bowl, start mixing everything with a spoon, then stir with your hands. Don't despair, the dough crumbles at first, but as it kneads it will be ready to shape. If the dough sticks to your hands, spread butter or water.
2. Take small portions, roll into balls, and then mash with a fork or spoon.
3. Bake for 8 minutes at 390°F in your deep fryer.

Nutrition Information

- Calories: 140
- Carbohydrates: 14g
- Fat: 8g
- Protein: 3g
- Sugar: 7g
- Cholesterol: 0mg

Banana Cookies

Servings: 7
Preparation time: 20 minutes
Cook time: 8 minutes

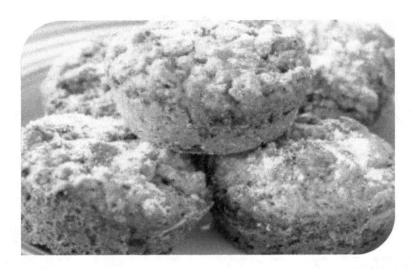

Ingredients

- 2 eggs
- ½ cup brown sugar
- 2 medium bananas
- ½ cup oven and stovetop sweetener
- ¼ cup coconut oil
- Cinnamon to taste
- 1 cup fine oat flakes
- ½ tbsp of baking powder

Steps to Cook

1. Put all the ingredients in the blender except the yeast.
2. Beat until smooth, add the yeast and mix with a spoon.
3. Distribute the dough leaving about 1 finger from the edge (so that the dough does not overflow).
4. Preheat your fryer for 5 minutes.
5. Take the cookies to the air fryer for 8 minutes at 350°F.

Nutrition Information

- Calories: 64.7
- Carbohydrates: 12.2g
- Fat: 1.8g
- Protein: 1.2g
- Sugar: 0.2g
- Cholesterol: 0mg

Pizza Fit

Servings: 4
Preparation time: 10 minutes
Cook time: 5 minutes

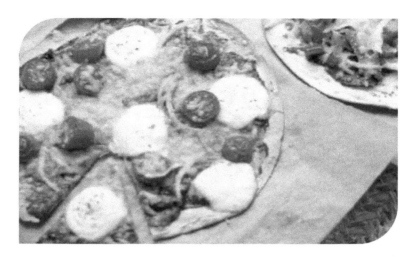

Ingredients

- 1 whole dough to wrap
- ½ tomato slices
- 2 slices of clear mozzarella
- homemade tomato sauce
- Shredded chicken to taste
- Olive oil to taste
- Oregano (optional)

Steps to Cook

1. Start by putting the sauce on the dough, then add the mozzarella, the chicken, lay out the tomato slices.
2. Sprinkle with oregano and drizzle with olive oil.
3. Preheat the electric fryer for 5 minutes.
4. Put the pizza already assembled and let it bake in the air fryer for 5 minutes at 350°F.

Nutrition Information

- Calories: 353
- Carbohydrates: 2g
- Fat: 13g
- Protein: 49g
- Sugar: 5g
- Cholesterol: 300mg

Bread Cake

Servings: 4-6
Preparation time: 5 minutes
Cook time: 15 minutes

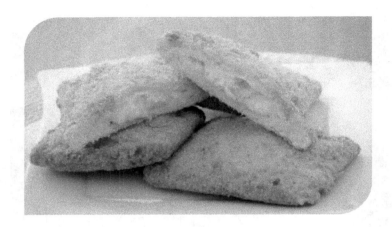

Ingredients

- 10 slices of bread without peel
- ½ lb of chopped cheese
- ½ lb minced ham
- oregano to taste
- 4 eggs
- Bread crumbs

Steps to Cook

1. Use the rolling pin and noodles to make the bread slices thinner or flatter;
2. Beat the eggs and reserve in powder.
3. Add a tablespoon of cheese, a tablespoon of ham and oregano;
4. Using a culinary brush, brush the beaten egg over the edges of the bread;
5. Using another slice of bread, cover the first and press the edges with a fork to close the cakes;
6. Repeat the procedure with the other cakes;
7. For the bread, first pass the cakes in the beaten egg and then in the breadcrumbs;
8. Place the cakes in the Air Fryer and fry them for 15 minutes at 350°F.

Nutrition Information

- Calories: 120
- Carbohydrates: 16g
- Fat: 5g
- Protein: 2g
- Sugar: 6g
- Cholesterol: 293mg

Onion Rings In Beer

Servings: 2-4
Preparation time: 5 minutes
Cook time: 15 minutes

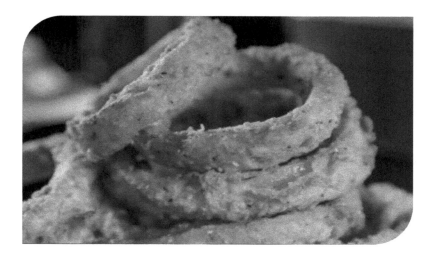

Ingredients

- 2 large onions cut into thick slices
- 1 can of beer at room temperature
- 1 cup of wheat flour
- Condiments to taste: such as condiments, chicken or beef broth, oregano, etc.
- Salt to taste

Steps to Cook

1. Mix all the ingredients until it turns into a not too smooth paste.
2. If necessary, use more flour or more beer until you get the point you need.
3. The rings must be completely covered with the dough before frying.
4. Put in the air fryer at 350°F for 15 minutes.
6. If the dough becomes too soft, it does not adhere properly to the onion rings.

Nutrition Information

- Calories: 410
- Carbohydrates: 45g
- Fat: 24g
- Protein: 3g
- Sugar: 5g
- Cholesterol: 0mg

Bread With Pepper And Garlic Confit

Servings: 40
Preparation time: 20 minutes
Cook time: 7 minutes

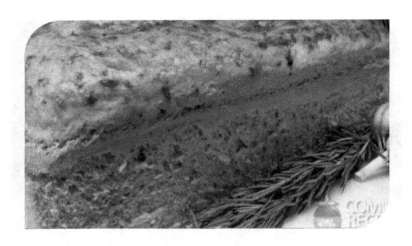

Ingredients

- 1 ½ cup of water
- 2 tbsp of yeast
- 1 spoon of sugar
- 1 egg
- 5 tbsp of piquet antipasto with garlic confit and habanero
- 3 ½ cups all-purpose flour
- 1 tbsp of salt

Steps to Cook

1. Put water, yeast and sugar in a bowl. Mix and let sit for 5 minutes, until the yeast begins to foam. Add the egg and antipasto and mix until smooth. Sift the flour, mix the salt and gradually add to the mixture, stirring until you can start kneading. On a smooth surface, add a little flour and start kneading.
2. Add a little flour and work the dough well so that the gluten develops well.
3. Grease the bread tray with oil and flour.
4. Lay out the dough, cover with a plastic film and let it rise for 45 minutes. Put in the air fryer preheated at 170°F, bake for 45 minutes. When removing, brush a little more of the antipasto on top to leave it with a very beautiful color.

Nutrition Information

- Calories: 350
- Carbohydrates: 32g
- Fat: 23g
- Protein: 6g
- Sugar: 2g
- Cholesterol: 0mg

Cocoa Bread

Servings: 12
Preparation time: 30 minutes
Cook time: 45 minutes

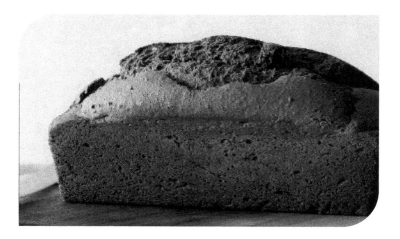

Ingredients

- ½ cup warm milk
- ½ cup coconut milk
- 3 tbsp of butter
- 4 tbsp of cocoa powder
- 1 tablet of fresh yeast
- 3 eggs
- 1 cup of sugar
- 4 ½ cups all-purpose flour
- Margarine fat

Topping:

½ lb dark chocolate
7 oz. milk cream

Steps to Cook

1. In a blender, mix the ingredients except the wheat flour.
2. In a bowl, add the beaten liquid with the flour and mix until smooth.
3. Knead the dough on a floured surface, leaving the dough soft and elastic.
4. Let stand for 30 minutes.
5. Roll the dough into a ball.
6. Place in a greased pan and place in the air fryer, preheated for 45 minutes.
7. Melt the chocolate in a bain-marie and mix with the cream.
8. Pour the icing on the hot bread. Serve immediately.

Nutrition Information

- Calories: 160
- Carbohydrates: 6g
- Fat: 12g
- Protein: 9g
- Sugar: 0g
- Cholesterol: 265mg

Quick Banana Bread

Servings: 10
Preparation time: 15 mins
Cook time: 35 minutes

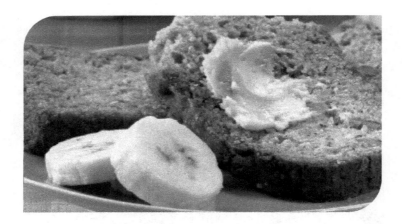

Ingredients

- ½ cup butter
- 1 cup of sugar
- 4 large mashed bananas
- ¼ cup milk
- 2 eggs
- 1 tbsp of vanilla sugar
- 1 tsp of baking soda
- 1 cup chopped chestnuts
- 1 tbsp baking powder
- 1 tbsp ground cinnamon
- 4 cups of flour

Steps to Cook

1. Mix all the ingredients and the flour, little by little until the point of dough similar to the cake dough, a little firmer.
2. Place in a bread pan, greased and sprinkled with wheat flour and bake in the air fryer at 350°F for browning, about 35 minutes.
3. Serve immediately.

Nutrition Information

- Calories: 195.6
- Carbohydrates: 32.8g
- Fat: 6.3g
- Protein: 2.6g
- Sugar: 5g
- Cholesterol: 25.8mg

Pullman Bread

Servings: 2-4
Preparation time: 15 minutes
Cook time: 30 minutes

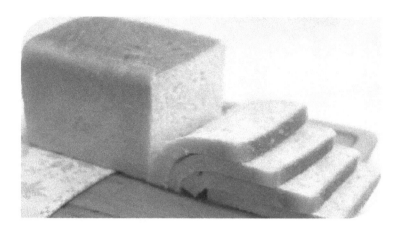

Ingredients

- 2 cups warm milk
- 1 tablet of yeast
- Wheat flour as enough
- 2 tbsp of sugar
- 1 egg
- 2 tbsp of olive oil
- 1 tbsp of margarine
- 1 pinch of salt

Steps to Cook

1. Dissolve the yeast in warm milk, add sugar and thicken with a little wheat flour.
2. Let it grow for 15 minutes.
3. Then mix the egg, oil, margarine, and salt.
4. Gradually add flour until it becomes a smooth dough.
5. Grease a baking sheet suitable for bread, pour the dough and let it rise on the baking sheet.
7. Put in the air fryer preheated at 350°F for 30 minutes or until golden.

Nutrition Information

- Calories: 2504
- Carbohydrates: 463.7g
- Fat: 32.2g
- Protein: 76.7g
- Sugar: 16.6g
- Cholesterol: 62mg

Onion Cream On Italian Bread

Servings: 8
Preparation time: 5 minutes
Cook time: 15 minutes

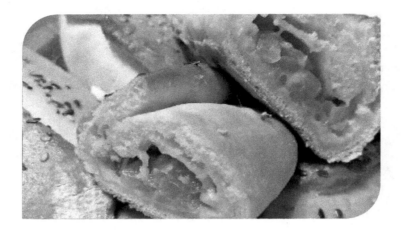

Ingredients

- 10 medium onions
- 2 ½ oz. of butter
- 1 oz. broth
- 8 ½ cups of water
- Wheat flour to taste
- Salt to taste
- Parmesan cheese for gratin

Steps to Cook

1. Sauté the onions in butter and fry them well.
2. Add the broth, flour and gradually add the water.
3. Cook well until thick.
4. Reservation.
5. Cut a lid off the Italian bread, remove the center and pour the cream inside.
6. Throw the Parmesan cheese on top. Put in the air fryer at 350°F for 15 minutes or until brown.
7. Serve immediately.

Nutrition Information

- Calories: 71
- Carbohydrates: 13.6g
- Fat: 0.87g
- Protein: 2.04g
- Sugar: 1.22g
- Cholesterol: 0mg

Pecan Pie With Breadcrumbs

Servings: 4-6
Preparation time: 10 minutes
Cook time: 20 minutes

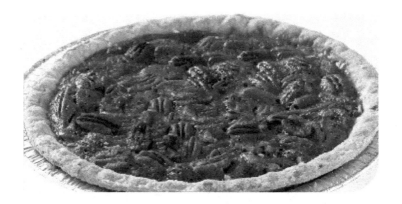

Ingredients

- ½ lb of coarsely chopped walnuts
- 6 eggs
- ½ lb of sugar
- 2 tbsp of breadcrumbs

Steps to Cook

1. Beat the egg whites in firm snow and set aside.
2. Beat the egg yolks with the very well beaten sugar.
3. Add the walnut kernels and bread crumbs.
4. Finally, add, simply by mixing, without beating, the egg whites.
5. The shape should be low, well greased with butter and lined with parchment paper also greased with moderate oven butter.
6. Put in the air fryer at 350°F for 20 minutes.
7. Once cooked, it can be covered with any cream.

Nutrition Information

- Calories: 380.9
- Carbohydrates: 57.7g
- Fat: 16.9g
- Protein: 3.7g
- Sugar: 48.6g
- Cholesterol: 53.6mg

Bread Cake With Apples And Dried Figs

Servings: 6-10
Preparation time: 7 minutes
Cook time: 15 minutes

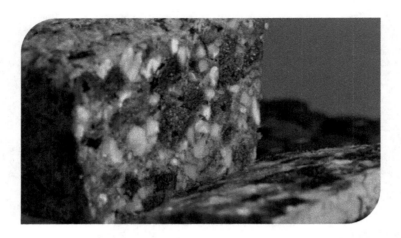

Ingredients

- ½ lb of chopped stale bread
- 2 cups of milk
- Peel ½ grated lemon
- 2 eggs
- ½ lb ricotta
- ½ cup of tea
- 5 apples
- 6 dried figs
- 1 pinch of salt
- 2 butter spoons
- 1 bunch of rosemary

Steps to Cook

1. Put the bread in a bowl. Add the hot milk and let it soften for 10 minutes. Then, knead with a fork until you get a homogeneous mixture. Add lemon peel, beaten eggs, ricotta cheese, sugar (reserve 2 tablespoons), 4 apples, peeled and diced, dried figs without petiole, chopped and without salt. Mix well until the dough is as homogeneous as possible. Line a 24cm x 36cm baking sheet with parchment paper. Pour the prepared dough and level the surface with a spatula. Cut the remaining apple in half, remove the seeds and cut it into 16 thin slices.
2. Using a knife, scratch the surface of the cake, dividing it into 16 pieces. Put an apple slice on each piece.
3. Spread the diced butter, rosemary, and remaining sugar on the surface of the cake. Put in the preheated air fryer at 350°F for 40 minutes.

Nutrition Information

- Calories: 278.2
- Carbohydrates: 58.8g
- Fat: 7.8g
- Protein: 3.3g
- Sugar: 42g
- Cholesterol: 10.8mg

Fried Yucca

Servings: 2-4
Preparation time: 5 minutes
Cook time: 1h 30 minutes

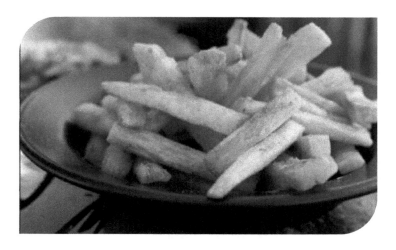

Ingredients

- 1 ¼ lb of cassava
- Salt to taste

Steps to Cook

1. Peel and cut the cassava in equal or as standardized sizes as possible.
2. After pressing the pan, leave your yucca in salted water for 10 minutes. Depending on the cassava, you will have to leave more time, check after 10 minutes if the cassava is soft enough to cut it, you need a cassava one point above the tooth.
3. Cut into strips or cubes according to your preference. Enjoy and remove the thick fibers of the cassava.
4. Drizzle a little olive oil, in addition to the flavor; it helps to color the cassava without leaving it dry and hard.
5. Preheat the deep fryer without oil for 3 minutes at 350°F.
6. Arrange the cassava in the basket; try to leave some passages free for air circulation.

Nutrition Information

- Calories: 152
- Carbohydrates: 28g
- Fat: 16g
- Protein: 1g

- Sugar: 1.2g
- Cholesterol: 0mg

Fried Plantain

Servings: 2-4
Preparation time: 5 minutes
Cook time: 9 minutes

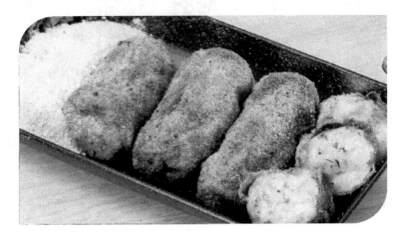

Ingredients

- 2 silver bananas
- 1 egg
- 4 ¼ oz. of breadcrumbs

Steps to Cook

1. Cutting the bananas in half is a good single serving. You can expand the recipe to the amount of bananas you want. There will be room in the fryer for at least 10 pieces of banana to fry.
2. Beat the whole egg well until smooth. Separate the bread crumbs into another container. Dip the banana in the egg and then roll it in breadcrumbs, squeeze so that the flour is put. Do this with all the pieces.
3. Preheat the fryer for 3 minutes at 400°F.
4. After that, put the pieces in the basket, avoiding touching them, no need to rotate, the Philips deep fryer fries all the parts very well. Fry for 9 minutes at 400°F. Notice the color that will be breading, gold and perfect.

Nutrition Information

- Calories: 64
- Carbohydrates: 11g
- Fat: 2g
- Protein: 0.4g
- Sugar: 5.9g
- Cholesterol: 0mg

Baked Cheese Bread

Servings: 2-4
Preparation time: 5 minutes
Cook time: 12 minutes

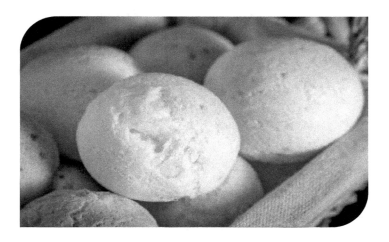

Ingredients

- ½ cup of oil
- ½ cup milk
- 2 eggs
- 1 ½ packet of sour powder
- ½ cup grated Parmesan cheese
- Salt to taste

Steps to Cook

1. Then, you will mix the oil, milk, and the two eggs in a blender (leave this mixture reserved in one corner). Take another bowl and add the starch to this mixture, plus the cheese and salt.
2. While preparing the dough, let your Air Fryer preheat for 5 minutes. Then, take the dough and place it in silicone molds ordering one next to the other. Allow another 7 minutes at 390°F.

Nutrition Information

- Calories: 71
- Carbohydrates: 12.52g
- Fat: 1.24g
- Protein: 2.21g
- Sugar: 1.07g
- Cholesterol: 1mg

Heart Of Palm Balls

Servings: 2-4
Preparation time: 5 minutes
Cook time: 15 minutes

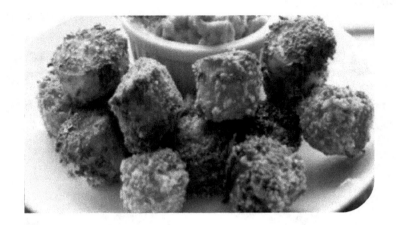

Ingredients

Mass:

- 1 pot of hearts of palm
- onion to taste
- 3 units of egg
- 3 stems of green chives
- 1 cup milk
- 3 ½ oz. of grated parmesan
- 1 tbsp baking powder
- 1 tbsp of salt
- 1 cup all-purpose flour

Steps to Cook

Mass:

1. Sauté the heart of palm with the onion.
2. In a bowl, place the heart of palm, eggs, chopped chives, cup of milk, grated Parmesan cheese.
3. Finally add the baking powder, salt and wheat flour.
4. Stir well to incorporate everything.
5. Place the dough in silicone molds and distribute it on the fryer tray.
6. Bake for 15 minutes at 350°F.

Nutrition Information

- Calories: 30
- Carbohydrates: 6g
- Fat: 0g
- Protein: 1g
- Sugar: 1g
- Cholesterol: 0mg

Breaded Camembert Cheese

Servings: 1-2
Preparation time: 5 minutes
Cook time: 15 minutes

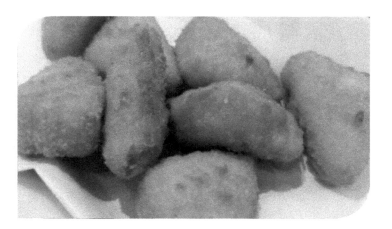

Ingredients

- 1 small camembert cheese
- 1 egg
- ½ cup breadcrumbs
- 2 tbsp of rice
- Honey or apricot jam to accompany

Steps to Cook

1. Beat the egg with a fork
2. Pass the camembert in the beaten egg and then in the breadcrumbs
3. Cover with parchment paper
4. Place the breaded cheese and drizzle with the olive oil.
5. Close the lid, set the cooking time to 15 minutes at 320^0F.
6. Serve hot with honey or jam.

Nutrition Information

- Calories: 242
- Carbohydrates: 10.4g
- Fat: 16.4g
- Protein: 12.2g
- Sugar: 0.6g
- Cholesterol: 35mg

Rye And Chorizo Bread

Servings: 2-4
Preparation time: 1h
Cook time: 20 minutes

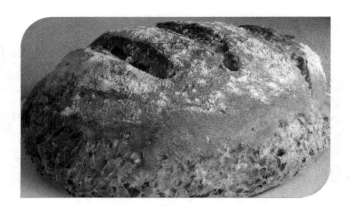

Ingredients

- 1 ¼ cup of water
- 1 lb wheat flour
- ¼ lb rye flour
- 1 tsp salty
- 1 ½ tsp yeast
- 4 slices of terra cheese
- chorizo meat

Steps to Cook

1. Premix the flours and stir a little to a deep plate to use later to sprinkle the bread.
2. Put the ingredients in the order as they are. At the end of the program, remove the dough and divide. Form a kind of semi-folded ball, pass the flour in the deep plate and place it in the fryer container.
3. Preheat the air fryer to 176°F for 1 minute. Allow it to cool slightly, and allow the bread to rise for approximately 1 hour before baking.
4. Meanwhile knead the remaining dough and divide it into 4 equal parts. With a rolling pin, roll each one into rectangles, place 1 slice of cheese in the middle of each one and fill with chorizo. Fold the sides and make some cuts on top, pass the rest of the flour and place on a baking sheet.
5. Put the bread inside and baked it for 20 minutes, after 10 minutes put aluminum foil on top. At the end it was cooled on a net, while baking the bread with chorizo, for 13 minutes at 350°F.

Nutrition Information

- Calories: 259
- Carbohydrates: 48g
- Fat: 3.3g
- Protein: 8.5g
- Sugar: 3.9g
- Cholesterol: 150mg

Sweet Fried Potatoes

Servings: 1-2
Preparation time: 5 minutes
Cook time: 15 minutes

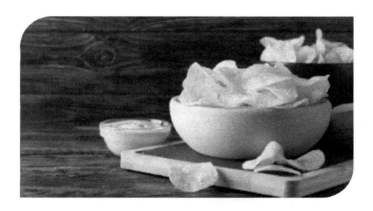

Ingredients

- 1 medium potato
- 1 olive oil bowl
- Salt to taste
- Oregano al gusto

Steps to Cook

1. Precooked potatoes
2. Cut into very thin slices.
3. Pass it in oil and sprinkle with salt.
4. Bake in the fryer for 15 minutes at 390°F. Avoid burn.
5. Serve with oregano.

Nutrition Information

- Calories: 149
- Carbohydrates: 12g
- Fat: 11g
- Protein: 0.8g
- Sugar: 3.1g
- Cholesterol: 0mg

Crispy Ham And Cheese Patty

Servings: 2-3
Preparation time: 5 minutes
Cook time: 7 minutes

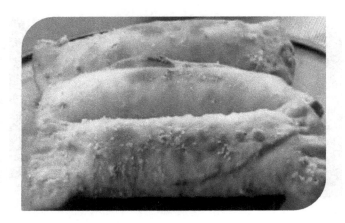

Ingredients

- *Pre-cooked lasagna dough (or puff pastry, the rectangular one)*
- *Sliced mozzarella cheese*
- *Sliced ham or turkey breast*
- *Tomato sauce or tomato sauce*
- *Mayonnaise*
- *Oregano*

Steps to Cook

1. In a rectangular dough (either lasagna or cake), place a tablespoon of tomato sauce or tomato sauce. Then add 1 slice of mozzarella and 1 slice of ham or turkey breast. Put 1 tablespoon of mayonnaise and spread it.
2. Carefully close the roll, like a cupcake. Using a fork, press down on the sides to close it firmly. To leave a golden cone, you will place 1 extra tablespoon of mayonnaise on top, spreading it over the entire surface.
3. Place in your air basket fryer for 7 minutes at 390°F. Then sprinkle more oregano and serve.

Nutrition Information

- Calories: 179.8
- Carbohydrates: 5g
- Fat: 17g
- Protein: 7g
- Sugar: 0g
- Cholesterol: 300mg

Pumpkin Cream On Italian Bread

Servings: 2-4
Preparation time: 5 minutes
Cook time: 10 minutes

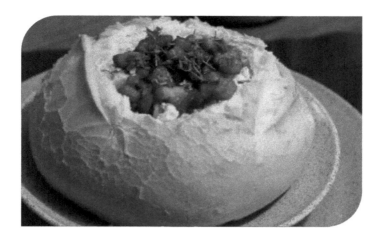

Ingredients

- 2 Italian loaves, round, medium
- 1 pound butternut squash
- 1 medium red onion, grated
- 1 garlic clove, crushed
- ½ lb of bacon
- 1 diced vegetable broth
- 1 cup chopped green tea
- 6 1/3 cups of water
- Parmesan to taste
- Salt and pepper

Steps to Cook

1. Cook the squash in the water with the vegetable bouillon cubes, until smooth.
2. In another skillet, sauté onion, garlic, and bacon in oil and separate.
3. Beat the pumpkin together with the cooking liquid in a blender or mixer (it is easier and produces less dirt), use the pan that removed the bacon and put the cream of whipped pumpkin, correct the salt if necessary
4. Put in the air fryer for 10 minutes at 320^0F sprinkled with green aroma to taste, bacon and parmesan.

Nutrition Information

- Calories: 200
- Carbohydrates: 31g
- Fat: 6g
- Protein: 5g
- Sugar: 9g
- Cholesterol: 285mg

Spring Roll

Servings: 4
Preparation time: 10 minutes
Cook time: 15 minutes

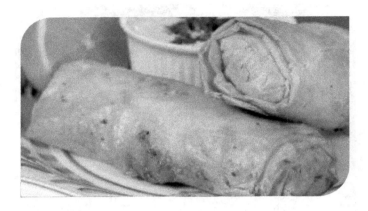

Ingredients

Mass:
- ½ lb of wheat flour
- 1 tbsp of oil
- 1 tbsp of salt
- ½ lb of water

Filling:
- ½ lb pork loin
- ½ lb cabbage
- 4 stems of green onion
- 1 tsp of ginger
- 1 tbsp of sake
- 2 tbsp of sesame oil
- Salt to taste

Steps to Cook

Filling:
1. In a saucepan, heat the sesame oil and fry the ground loin. Add sake and salt (optional). Cook for a few minutes. Add the chopped cabbage and grated ginger.
2. Cook until cabbage wilts. Add the chives. Stir and turn off. Reserve.

Mass:
3. In a bowl, place the flour, salt, oil (optional) and water, little by little, always stirring. Heat a round, nonstick skillet. Roll out portions of the dough with the help of a brush. Remove when not glued from the pan.
1. Then fill and roll. Glue the tip with a little raw dough.
2. Put in the air fryer at $350°F$ for 15 minutes.

Nutrition Information

- Calories: 170
- Carbohydrates: 70g
- Fat: 0g
- Protein: 16g
- Sugar: 38g
- Cholesterol: 210mg

Palmetto

Servings: 4-8
Preparation time: 5 minutes
Cook time: 10 minutes

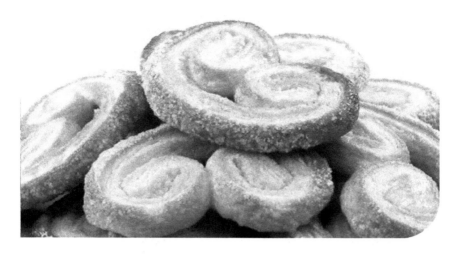

Ingredients

- ½ lb puff pastry
- ¼ lb of palm heart
- 1 tomato
- 1 ½ oz. of mozzarella cheese
- ½ cup of warm water
- 1 yolk
- Oregano to taste
- Salt to taste
- Black pepper to taste

Steps to Cook

1. Cut the dough as you like.
2. Chop the heart of palm, tomato and mozzarella cheese.
3. Add oregano, salt and pepper according to your preference.
4. Fill and seal the dough with a fork.
5. Preheat the air fryer for 5 minutes, adjusting the temperature to 350°F.
6. Place the puff pastry in the cooking basket.
7. Set the timer to 10 minutes.
8. Remove and serve while still hot

Nutrition Information

- Calories: 140
- Carbohydrates: 1g
- Fat: 13g
- Protein: 4g
- Sugar: 4g
- Cholesterol: 280mg

Croque Monsieur

Servings: 4
Preparation time: 5 minutes
Cook time: 2 minutes

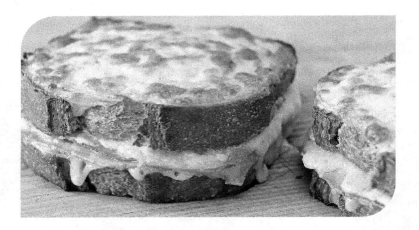

Ingredients

- 8 slices of white bread, shelled
- 4 slices of lean ham
- 4 slices of mozzarella cheese
- 1 ½ oz. of mozzarella cheese
- 1 tbsp of flour
- 1 tbsp butter
- ¼ cup milk

Steps to Cook

1. Assemble the sandwiches with ham and cheese.
2. In a saucepan melt the butter and place the flour. Stir with a source until golden. Add the milk and stir until it forms a thick sauce. Season the bechamel sauce with salt and pepper to taste.
3. Place a slice of cheese on top of each sandwich and the bechamel sauce.
4. Preheat the appliance for 5 minutes, adjusting the temperature to 390°F.
5. Place the sandwiches in the cooking basket at least 2 cm apart.
6. Between them and the walls of the inner tray.
7. Set the timer to 3 minutes.
8. Remove and serve while still hot.

Nutrition Information

- Calories: 282
- Carbohydrates: 21g
- Fat: 14g
- Protein: 15g
- Sugar: 1g
- Cholesterol: 276mg

Bread Gnocchi

Servings: 20
Preparation time: 5 minute
Cook time: 35 minutes

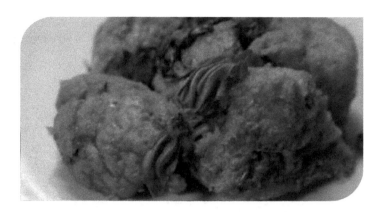

Ingredients

- 1 lb of stale bread
- ½ liter of milk
- 2 tbsp olive oil
- ½ lb of bacon cut into strips
- 3 ½ oz. of wheat flour
- 2 eggs
- 4 tbsp grated cheese
- 1 tbsp chopped parsley
- 1 ½ oz. of butter
- Salt to taste
- 1 tbsp parsley for decoration

Steps to Cook

1. Break and let the bread soak in the milk. Let water, strain and squeeze well. Brown the bacon at 350°F for 15 minutes. Set aside.
2. In a bowl, mix together bread, three tablespoons of wheat flour, eggs, and two tablespoons of grated cheese, parsley and drained bacon.
3. Form balls into quail eggs.
4. Boil plenty of salted water and place the floured gnocchi.
5. When they rise to the surface, scoop them out.
6. Season with melted butter and the rest of the grated cheese.
7. Garnish with bacon and parsley.

Nutrition Information

- Calories: 254
- Carbohydrates: 52g
- Fat: 1.5g
- Protein: 7.7g
- Sugar: 0.8g
- Cholesterol: 37mg

Chapter 4

Air Fryer Poultry Recipes

Chicken Meatballs

Servings: 2
Preparation time: 5 minutes
Cook time: 15 minutes

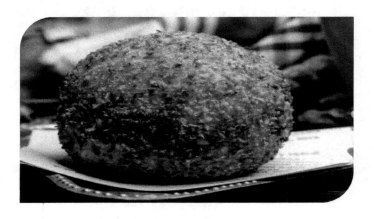

Ingredients

- ½ lb chicken breast
- 1 tbsp of garlic
- 1 tbsp of onion
- ½ chicken broth
- 1 tbsp of oatmeal, whole wheat flour or of your choice
- 1 pinch of paprika
- Salt and black pepper

Steps to Cook

1. Put all ingredients in a food processor and beat well until well mixed and ground.
2. If you don't have a food processor, ask the butcher to grind it and then add the other ingredients, mixing well.
3. Make balls and place them in the Air Fryer basket.
4. Program the Air Fryer for 15 minutes at 400°F.
5. Half the time shake the basket so that the meatballs loosen and fry evenly..

Nutrition Information

- Calories: 45
- Carbohydrates: 1.94g
- Fat: 1.57g
- Protein: 5.43g
- Sugar: 0.41g
- Cholesterol: 23m

Homemade Breaded Nugget In Doritos

Servings: 4
Preparation time: 10 minutes
Cook time: 15 minutes

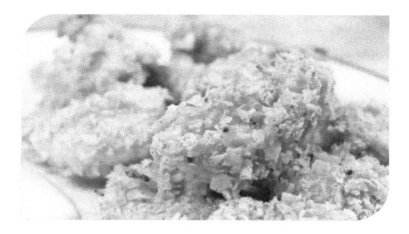

Ingredients

- ½ lb boneless, skinless chicken breast
- ¼ lb Doritos snack
- 1 cup of wheat flour
- 1 egg
- Salt, garlic and black pepper to taste.

Steps to Cook

1. Cut the chicken breast in the width direction, 1 to 1.5 cm thick, so that it is already shaped like pips.
2. Season with salt, garlic, black pepper to taste and some other seasonings if desired.
3. You can also season with those seasonings or powdered onion soup.
4. Put the Doritos snack in a food processor or blender and beat until everything is crumbled, but don't beat too much, you don't want flour.
5. Now bread, passing the pieces of chicken breast first in the wheat flour, then in the beaten eggs and finally in the Doritos, without leaving the excess flour, eggs or Doritos.
6. Place the seeds in the Air Fryer basket and program for 15 minutes at 400°F, and half the time they brown evenly.

Nutrition Information

- Calories: 42
- Carbohydrates: 1.65g
- Fat: 1.44g
- Protein: 5.29g
- Sugar: 0.1g
- Cholesterol: 20mg

Chicken Breast

Servings: 6
Preparation time: 30 minutes
Cook time: 25 minutes

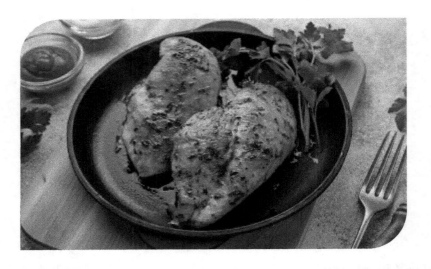

Ingredients

- 1 lb diced clean chicken breast
- ½ lemon
- Smoked paprika to taste
- Black pepper or chili powder, to taste
- Salt to taste

Steps to Cook

1. Season the chicken with salt, paprika and pepper and marinate.
2. Store in Air fryer and turn on for 15 minutes at 350°F.
3. Turn the chicken over and raise the temperature to 200°C, and turn the Air Fryer on for another 5 minutes or until golden.
4. Serve immediately.

Nutrition Information

- Calories: 124
- Carbohydrates: 0g
- Fat: 1.4g
- Protein: 26.1g
- Sugar: 0g
- Cholesterol: 66mg

Homemade Chicken Nuggets

Servings: 4
Preparation time: 30 minutes
Cook time: 15 minutes

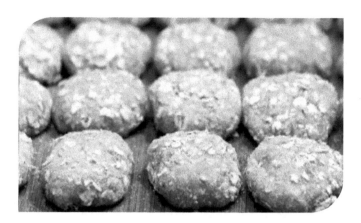

Ingredients

- 1 lb of chicken breast
- 1 large onion
- 2 garlic cloves
- Marjoram to taste (leaves only)
- Salt and pepper

To the bread:

- Bread crumbs
- Oatmeal
- Hot paprika
- Wheat flour
- 3 eggs
- Salt

Steps to Cook

1. In the food processor, place the chicken into pieces, the onion broken into 6 parts, the garlic, the marjoram leaves, salt and pepper. Whisk until the dough is smooth and even.
2. Roll the chicken dough into balls and place them on a tray, using 15 g of chicken paste as standard so that the seeds are similar in size.
3. Now prepare the ingredients for breading. In a bowl mix a part of oatmeal with a part of breadcrumbs and season with a little paprika, in the second bowl put the flour and in a third bowl break the eggs, add salt and put a few tablespoons of water to leave the mixture it is less thick and therefore increases performance.
4. Now it's time for bread, roll the chicken ball in the egg, then in the white flour, return to the egg and pass the mixture of oatmeal and breadcrumbs.
5. At this point, you will form the nuggets, leaving them with a rectangular shape, but not with perfect shapes.
6. Put it in the air fryer for 30 minutes at 400^0F.

Nutrition Information

- Calories: 215.6
- Carbohydrates: 9.9g
- Fat: 13.4g
- Protein: 13g
- Sugar: 0.2g
- Cholesterol: 96.4

Breaded Chicken Without Flour

Servings: 6
Preparation time: 10 minutes
Cook time: 15 minutes

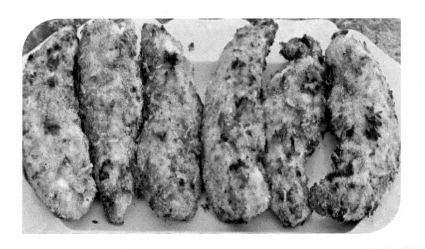

Ingredients

- 1 1/6 oz. of grated parmesan cheese
- 1 unit of egg
- 1 lb of chicken (breast)
- Salt to taste
- To taste black pepper

Steps to Cook

7.
1. Cut the chicken breast into 6 fillets and season with a little salt and pepper.
2. Beat the egg in a bowl.
3. Pass the chicken breast in the egg and then in the grated cheese, sprinkling the fillets.
4. Non-stick and put in the air fryer at 400°F for about 30 minutes or until golden brown.

Nutrition Information

- Calories: 114
- Carbohydrates: 13g
- Fat: 5.9g
- Protein: 2.3g
- Sugar: 3.2g
- Cholesterol: 19mg

Buffalo Wings

Servings: 2
Preparation time: 5 minutes
Cook time: 30-35 minutes

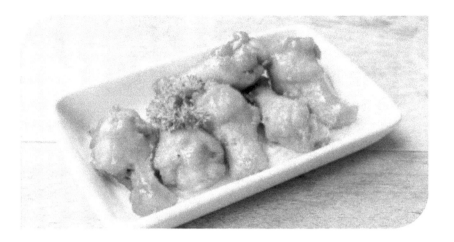

Ingredients

Wings:
- 2 pounds chicken wings
- 1 tbsp avocado oil
- ½ tsp garlic powder
- ½ tsp salt
- extra oil to grease
- 1/3 cup hot pepper

Sauce:
- ¼ cup butter
- 1 tbsp of white vinegar
- 1/8 tsp of pepper

Steps to Cook

Wings:
1. In a large bowl, accept olive oil in pollen and warm sprays and add octopus and salt. Jar into the fryer basket with a little more olive oil, avocado oil, and coconut oil. Place the pollen bags on a single cover in the basket. Cook the wings at 360°F for 25 minutes.
2. Go back to the wings. Then increase the temperature to 400°F and cook for 4 more minutes.

Sauce:
3. Put the hot sauce, butter, vinegar, and hot pepper in a small bowl. Let it boil over medium heat and beat it. Set it aside. When the wings are done, add the sauce and cover. Serve with blue cheese.

Nutrition Information

- Calories: 70
- Carbohydrates: 0g
- Fat: 5g
- Protein: 6g
- Sugar: 0g
- Cholesterol: 25mg

Barbecue With Chorizo and Chicken

Servings: 1-4
Preparation time: 5 minutes
Cook time: 35 minutes

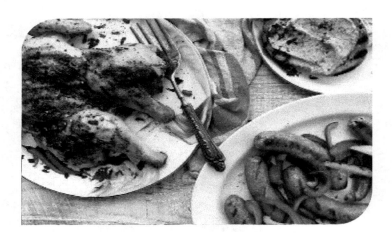

Ingredients

- 4 chicken thighs
- 2 Tuscan sausages
- 4 small onions

Steps to Cook

1. Preheat the fryer to 400°F for 5 minutes. Season the meat the same way you would if you were going to use the barbecue.
2. Put in the fryer, lower the temperature to 160°C and set for 30 minutes.
3. After 20 minutes, check if any of the meat has reached the point of your preference. If so, take whichever is ready and return to the fryer with the others for another 10 minutes, now at 400°F. If not, return them to Air Fryer for the last 10 minutes at 400°F.

Nutrition Information

- Calories: 135
- Carbohydrates: 0g
- Fat: 5g
- Protein: 6g
- Sugar: 0g
- Cholesterol: 300mg

Roasted Thigh

Servings: 1
Preparation time: 5 minutes
Cook time: 30 minutes

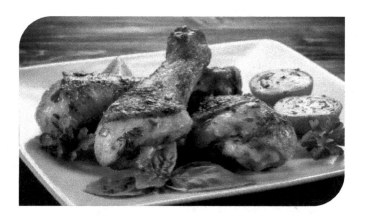

Ingredients

- 3 chicken thighs and thighs
- 2 red seasonal bags
- 1 clove garlic
- ½ tsp of salt
- 1 pinch of black pepper

Steps to Cook

1. Season chicken with red season, minced garlic, salt, and pepper. Leave to act for 5-10 minutes to obtain the flavor.
2. Place the chicken in the Air Fryer basket and bake at 390°F for 20 minutes.
3. After that time, remove the Air Fryer basket and check the chicken spot. If it is still raw or not golden enough, turn it over and leave it for another 10 minutes at 350°F.
4. After the previous step, your chicken will be ready on the Air Fryer! Serve with doré potatoes and leaf salad.

Nutrition Information

- Calories: 278
- Carbohydrates: 0.1g
- Fat: 18g
- Protein: 31g
- Sugar: 0g
- Cholesterol: 166mg

Hot Smoked Wings

Servings: 4-6
Preparation time: 10 mins
Cook time: 17 minutes

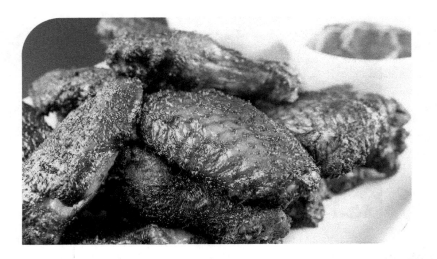

Ingredients

- 2 ¼ lb chicken wings
- ½ chopped onion
- 5 cloves garlic, minced
- 2 tbsp of smoked paprika
- 2 tbsp of hot paprika
- 1 tbsp of cayenne pepper
- Salt
- black pepper to taste
- ½ lb of wheat
- ½ cup of beer
- 1 tbsp of baking soda

Steps to Cook

1. Season the chicken with salt and pepper and set aside.
2. Mix the onion, garlic, paprika and cayenne pepper until it becomes a homogeneous mass.
3. Add wheat, baking soda, and beer to a very pasty paste.
4. It can't be too liquid so it doesn't crumble in the fryer.
5. Dip the wings in the dough until they are completely covered, that is, with the chicken covered with the dough.
6. Fry in the fryer at 350°F for 17 minutes.
7. Serve with your favorite sauce like barbecue, tomato sauce, or blue cheese with garlic.

Nutrition Information

- Calories: 530
- Carbohydrates: 5g
- Fat: 40g
- Protein: 36g
- Sugar: 2g
- Cholesterol: 155mg

Coxinha Fit

Servings: 2-4
Preparation time: 10 minutes
Cook time: 10-15 minutes

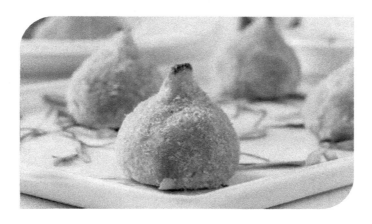

Ingredients

- ½ lb seasoned and minced chicken
- 1 cup light cottage cheese
- 1 egg
- Condiments to taste
- Flaxseed or oatmeal

Steps to Cook

1. Mix all ingredients together in a bowl except flour.
2. Knead well with your hands and mold into coxinha format.
3. If you prefer you can fill it, add chicken or cheese.
4. Repeat the process until all the dough is gone.
5. Pass the drumsticks in the flour and put them in the fryer.
6. Bake for 10 to 15 minutes at 390°F or until golden.
7. Now it only works!

Nutrition Information

- Calories: 220
- Carbohydrates: 40g
- Fat: 18g
- Protein: 100g
- Sugar: 5g
- Cholesterol: 3000mg

Rolled Turkey Breast

Servings: 4
Preparation time: 5 minutes
Cook time: 10 minutes

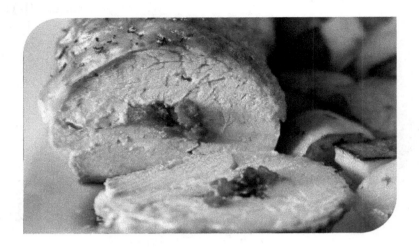

Ingredients

- 1 box of cherry tomatoes
- ¼ lb turkey blanket

Steps to Cook

1. Wrap the turkey and blanket in the tomatoes, close with the help of toothpicks.
2. Take to Air Fryer for 10 minutes at 390°F.
3. You can increase the filling with ricotta and other preferred light ingredients.

Nutrition Information

- Calories: 172
- Carbohydrates: 3g
- Fat: 2g
- Protein: 34g
- Sugar: 1g
- Cholesterol: 300mg

Chicken In Beer

Servings: 4
Preparation time: 5 minutes
Cook time: 10 minutes

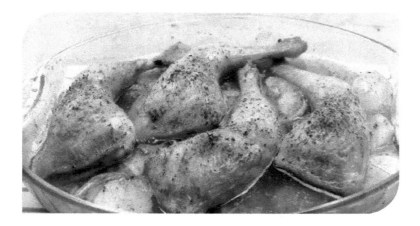

Ingredients

- 2 ¼ lbs chicken thigh and thigh
- ½ can of beer
- 4 cloves of garlic
- 1 large onion
- Pepper and salt to taste

Steps to Cook

1. Wash the chicken pieces and, if desired, remove the skin to be healthier.
2. Place on an ovenproof plate.
3. In the blender, beat the other ingredients: beer, onion, garlic, and add salt and pepper, all together.
4. Cover the chicken with this mixture; it has to stay like swimming in the beer.
5. Take to the preheated air fryer at 390°F for 45 minutes.
6. It will roast when it has a brown cone on top and the beer has dried a bit.

Nutrition Information

- Calories: 674
- Carbohydrates: 5.47g
- Fat: 41.94g
- Protein: 61.94g
- Sugar: 1.62g
- Cholesterol: 206mg

Chicken Fillet

Servings: 2-4
Preparation time: 5 minutes
Cook time: 20 minutes

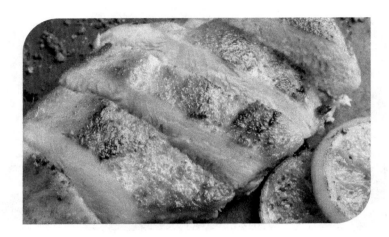

Ingredients

- 4 chicken fillets
- salt to taste
- 1 garlic clove, crushed
- thyme to taste
- black pepper to taste

Steps to Cook

1. Add seasoning to fillets, wrapping well for flavor. Preheat the Air Fryer for 5 minutes at 350°F. Place the fillets in the basket, program for 20 minutes at 350°F. With 5 minutes remaining, turn the fillets and raise the temperature to 390°F. Serve!

Nutrition Information

- Calories: 90
- Carbohydrates: 1g
- Fat: 1g
- Protein: 17g
- Sugar: 0g
- Cholesterol: 45mg

Chicken Thigh With Potatoes

Servings: 2-4
Preparation time: 30 minutes
Cook time: 30 minutes

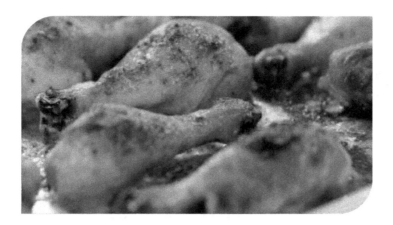

Ingredients

- 1 lb of chicken on the thighs;
- 1 tbsp crushed garlic;
- 1 tsp of paprika;
- 1 tsp of vinegar;
- 1 tbsp of olive oil;
- salt to taste;
- Black pepper to taste

Potatoes:

- 3 medium potatoes;
- 1 tbsp of olive oil;
- herbs to taste;
- salt to taste;
- black pepper to taste.

Steps to Cook

1. In a plastic bowl or seasoning bag, place the chicken seasonings and help. Marinate for 30 minutes or more for flavor.
2. In another container, place the potatoes, peeled and cut into 4 cm pieces. Season well and let it rest, too.
3. Place the potatoes in the bottom of the Air Fryer basket and place the previously marinated chickens on top.
4. Set for 15 minutes at 390^0F. After that time, turn the chicken over and leave for another 15 minutes or until golden brown to your liking. Serve!

Nutrition Information

- Calories: 135
- Carbohydrates: 0g
- Fat: 8.45g
- Protein: 13.67g
- Sugar: 0g
- Cholesterol: 51mg

Chicken Wings With Mustard

Servings: 2-4
Preparation time: 30 mins
Cook time: 300 minutes

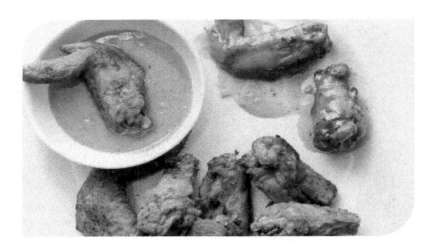

Ingredients

- 2 ¼ lb chicken wing
- 1 onion
- 2 lemons squeezed;
- 2 tbsp of mustard;
- 2 tbsp of parsley;
- 2 tbsp grated Parmesan;
- 3 garlic cloves;
- salt to taste;
- Black pepper to taste.

Steps to Cook

1. Put the onion, lemon juice and mustard in a blender and mix for 1 minute. Add parsley, garlic, and Parmesan and beat for another minute.
2. Season the sauce with salt and pepper to taste.
3. Put the sauce on the chicken wings and put it well. Let it marinate for 30 minutes.
4. Place the chicken in the Air Fryer basket at 390°F and cook for 15 minutes, reserving the rest of the sauce. Flip the chicken over. Add the rest of the sauce and leave for another 15 minutes. Serve!

Nutrition Information

- Calories: 550
- Carbohydrates: 36g
- Fat: 40g
- Protein: 40g
- Sugar: 5g
- Cholesterol: 36mg

Chicken With Lemon And Bahian Seasoning

Servings: 2-4
Preparation time: 2h
Cook time: 20 minutes

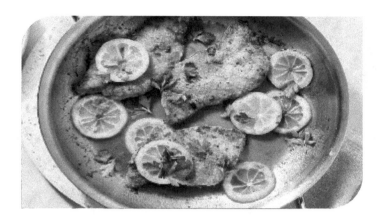

Ingredients

- 5 pieces of chicken to bird;
- 2 garlic cloves, crushed;
- 4 tablespoons of lemon juice;
- 1 coffee spoon of Bahian spices;
- salt to taste;
- Black pepper to taste.

Steps to Cook

1. Place the chicken pieces in a covered bowl and add the spices. Add the lemon juice. Cover the container and let the chicken marinate for 2 hours.
2. Place each piece of chicken in the basket of the electric fryer, without overlapping the pieces. Set the fryer for 20 minutes at 390°F. In half the time, brown evenly. Serve!

Nutrition Information

- Calories: 316.2
- Carbohydrates: 4.9g
- Fat: 15.3g
- Protein: 32.8g
- Sugar: 0g
- Cholesterol: 0mg

Whole Chicken

Servings: 2-4
Preparation time: 5 minutes
Cook time: 25 minutes

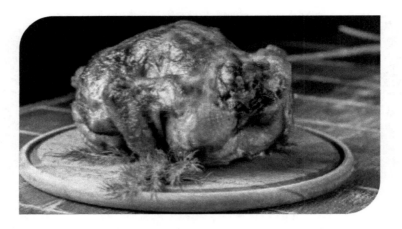

Ingredients

- 1 clean whole chicken;
- 1 small green bell pepper, chopped;
- 1 tbsp of salt;
- 2 cloves crushed garlic
- 1 bunch of chopped parsley;
- 1 tsp of paprika;
- 5 chopped bay leaves;
- 2 medium chopped onions;
- Light chicken broth;
- ¼ cup of dry white wine.

Steps to Cook

1. In a blender, mix all the ingredients. Pass the blender mixture over the chicken, inside and out.
2. Place the chicken in a bag with the seasoning and marinate overnight for flavor.
3. The next day, remove the chicken from the envelope and discard the remaining seasoning. Place chicken in Air Fryer basket with breast side down.
4. Set your Air Fryer for 20 minutes at 390^0F.
5. After that time, turn the chicken over and adjust for another 20 minutes at 390°F. Serve!

Nutrition Information

- Calories: 1429
- Carbohydrates: 0g
- Fat: 81g
- Protein: 163g
- Sugar: 0g
- Cholesterol: 526m

Chicken Fingers

Servings: 2-4
Preparation time: 30 minutes
Cook time: 25 minutes

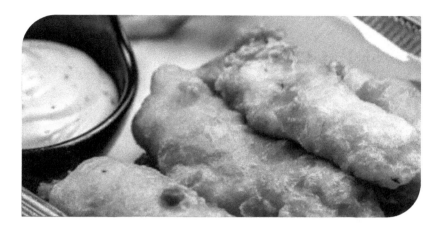

Ingredients

- 6 chicken breast fillets
- 1 garlic clove, finely minced
- salt to taste
- lemon drops
- black pepper to taste
- oatmeal
- cassava flour
- Olive oil

Steps to Cook

1. Season the chicken fillets and marinate for 30 minutes and collect the flavors.
2. In a plate, place the flours and bread the fillets. Reservation. Preheat your Air Fryer for 10 minutes at 390°F.
3. Then place the fillets and set for 15 minutes at 350°F. If you still want crispier, come back for longer. Serve.

Nutrition Information

- Calories: 112
- Carbohydrates: 7.1g
- Fat: 6.2g
- Protein: 7g
- Sugar: 0.1g
- Cholesterol: 17mg

Chapter 5

Air Fryer Meat (Beef, Pork and Lamb) Recipes

Interior Pork Rib

Servings: 6-8
Preparation time: 15 minutes
Cook time: 50-60 minutes

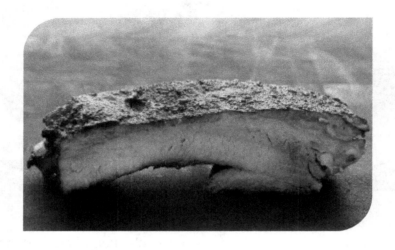

Ingredients

- 4 ½ lbs of pork ribs
- 1 tbsp of oil
- 2 tbsp of chopped onion
- ½ cup brown sugar
- ½ cup white vinegar
- 2 tbsp Worcestershire sauce
- 2 cups tomato sauce
- 1 bay leaf
- 1 tbsp of chili powder
- ½ cup of water
- Salt and black pepper
  - 2 broth broth tablets

Steps to Cook

1. Spread the salt over all the meat and boil for 5 minutes in a pan with plenty of hot water with 2 broth tablets. Drain the water.
2. Place the ribs on a baking sheet, cover with aluminum foil and put in the air fryer for 30 minutes at 400°F.
3. In a saucepan, sauté the onion in the oil, add the brown sugar and vinegar, and allow the sugar to dissolve. Add Worcestershire sauce, tomato sauce, bay leaf, chili powder and water and cook for 10 minutes or until sauce thickens.
4. Spice with salt and pepper.
5. After 30 minutes, remove the ribs from the air fryer, remove the foil and brush with the sauce.
16. Bake the ribs for another 10 minutes, brush with the sauce, and bake for another 5 minutes and repeat this operation again.

Nutrition Information

- Calories: 270
- Carbohydrates: 0g
- Fat: 21g
- Protein: 19g
- Sugar: 2g
- Cholesterol: 75mg

Elegant Interior Ribs

Servings: 6-8
Preparation time: 15 minutes
Cook time: 50-60 minutes

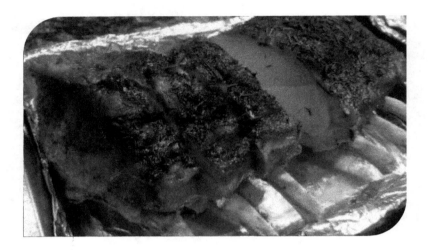

Ingredients

- 4 ½ lbs of pork ribs
- 1 lemon juice
- Salt to taste
- 3 garlic cloves
- Ground pepper to taste

Sauce:

- 2 tbsp of honey
- 2 tbsp soy sauce
- 2 tbsp Worcestershire sauce
- 2 tbsp of brown sugar
- 2 tbsp of mustard
- 2 cups tomato sauce
- 1 glass of water
- Salt to taste

Steps to Cook

1. Season the ribs with squeezed garlic, salt, lemon and Worcestershire sauce.
2. In a bowl, mix the sauce ingredients and reserve.
3. Before taking it to the air fryer, place the ribs in a pan with boiling water to remove excess fat.
4. Very fast, just a slight boil. Spread some oil on a baking sheet and place the ribs. Also add 3 whole onions, 4 chopped potatoes and 2 garlic heads.
5. Cover with aluminum foil and put it in the air fryer at 400°F for 40 minute.
6. After that time, cook the potatoes, onions, and garlic. Then take it out of the air fryer and set it aside. Remove the paper and let the ribs bake a little longer.
7. Put half of the sauce and leave it for another 15 minutes. At that time, it is worth trying the meat to feel if it is already tender.
8. In the last minutes, put the rest of the sauce so that it does not dry completely.

Nutrition Information

- Calories: 270
- Carbohydrates: 0g
- Fat: 21g
- Protein: 19g
- Sugar: 2g
- Cholesterol: 75mg

Stuffed Loin

Servings: 4
Preparation time: 20 minutes
Cook time: 40 minutes

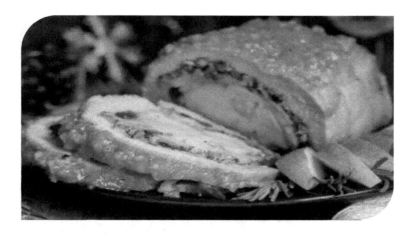

Ingredients

- 1 ¼ lbs of pork loin
- 1 tbsp of olive oil
- 1 tbsp crushed garlic
- 1 tbsp of vinegar
- 1 pinch of paprika
- Salt and black pepper
- Rosemary (optional)

Filling:

- ½ slice of smoked sausage
- 2 slices of fresh Tuscan sausage
- 1 cup prepared farofa

Steps to Cook

1. Lay the loin on a meat cutting board, and with a sharp knife open it like a blanket, like cutting meat to open and roll. Season the loin with olive oil, garlic, vinegar, salt and pepper. Then put the crushed or finely chopped pepperoni sausage in a bowl, remove the skin from the fresh Tuscan sausages and add the prepared flour, mix well, it will turn into a raw flour.
2. Now place this farofa on the spine, distribute and press to paste, leave about 3 fingers without filling so that you can close at the end.
3. Roll the loin like a roll and glue some toothpicks at the end to hold the tip.
4. Put the sirloin in the basket of the Air Fryer. Adjust the Air Fryer for 40 minutes at 400°F. At this point, the tenderloin is ready and at the correct point.

Nutrition Information

- Calories: 296
- Carbohydrates: 4g
- Fat: 16g
- Protein: 32g
- Sugar: 0g
- Cholesterol: 211mg

Kafta

Servings: 8
Preparation time: 10 minutes
Cook time: 20 minutes

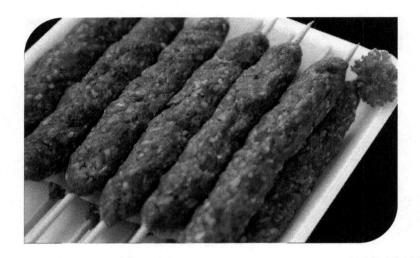

Ingredients

- ½ lb of ground meat
- 3 tbsp finely chopped onion
- 1 tbsp crushed garlic
- 2 to 3 tbsp of parsley
- Salt to taste
- 1 tbsp of Syrian pepper
- 8 skewers that fit in the Air Fryer, if they are large, break one piece of each to fit

Steps to Cook

1. Put all the ingredients in a bowl and mix well, then divide them into 8 equal parts and form the skewers forming the kafta.
2. Place the organized skewers inside the Air Fryer basket so that the hot air can circulate, as in the images below, then program for 20 minutes at 400°F, turning the skewers in half this time.
3. If you like it weirder, leave less time.

Nutrition Information

- Calories: 221
- Carbohydrates: 2g
- Fat: 7g
- Protein: 34g
- Sugar: 0g
- Cholesterol: 199mg

Pork Tenderloin With Mustard And Honey

Servings: 2
Preparation time: 10 minutes
Cook time: 15 minutes

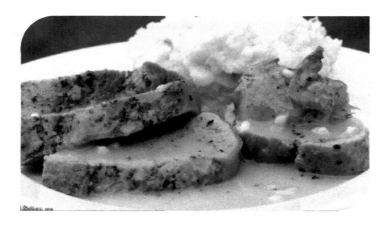

Ingredients

- 1 lb of pork fillet
- 1 tbsp of mustard
- 1 tbsp of honey
- 1 tbsp of lemon juice or vinegar
- ½ tsp salt
- 1 tsp crushed garlic
- 1 pinch of black pepper

Steps to Cook

1. Cut or ask the butcher to cut the fillets to a thickness of at least 1 cm.
2. In a small bowl mix all the ingredients and make a sauce, then roll out the fillets, brushing on both sides.
3. Place as many fillets in the preheated Air Fryer basket and adjust for 10 minutes at 400°F.
4. After this time, brush the fillets again with the rest of the sauce and turn them over, set another 5 minutes at 400°F and serve.

Nutrition Information

- Calories: 130
- Carbohydrates: 11g
- Fat: 2g
- Protein: 17g
- Sugar: 7g
- Cholesterol: 50mg

Picanha In Bread Bag

Servings: 2
Preparation time: 30 minutes
Cook time: 90 minutes

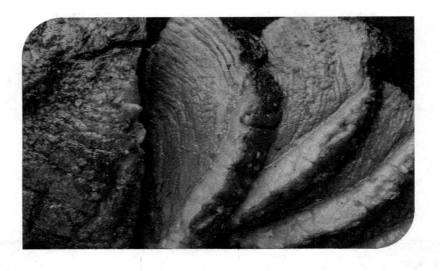

Ingredients

- 2 lbs Picanha
- 2 lbs coarse salt
- 3 ½ oz. margarine
- 1 bag of bread (paper) containing the picanha

Steps to Cook

1. Pass the margarine throughout the paper bag, evenly.
2. Cover the bottom of the paper bag with a portion of the coarse salt.
3. Place the picanha with the fat on top and cover with the remaining coarse salt.
4. Fill the bag with air and close it with a string.
5. After an hour in the air fryer at 400°F, remove the steak from the bag and return to the air fryer to brown.

Nutrition Information

- Calories: 390
- Carbohydrates: 1.3g
- Fat: 24g
- Protein: 42g
- Sugar: 0g
- Cholesterol: 135mg

Meatballs

Servings: 4-6
Preparation time: 5 minutes
Cook time: 15 minutes

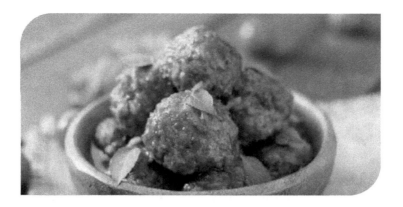

Ingredients

- ½ lb of ground meat
- 1 garlic clove, crushed
- ¼ of onion chopped
- 2 tbsp green smell
- 1 tsp of paprika or paprika
- ½ package of meat broth powder (optional)
- Salt and black pepper

Steps to Cook

1. In a bowl, mix all the ingredients and knead well with your hands, to make it an even mixture.
2. Mold the mixture into a ball and place it directly into the fryer basket.
3. Set the machine for 15 minutes at 400°F.
4. Half the time, shake the air fryer basket so that the meatballs brown evenly.

Nutrition Information

- Calories: 300
- Carbohydrates: 19g
- Fat: 18g
- Protein: 13g
- Sugar: 6g
- Cholesterol: 35mg

Breaded Suckling Pig Fillet

Servings: 4
Preparation time: 30 minutes
Cook time: 25 minutes

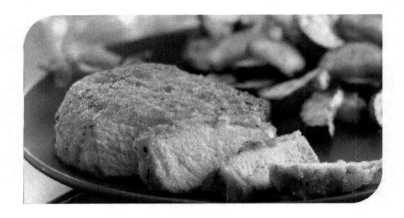

Ingredients

- 1 ½ lb of pork fillet
- 2 cups milk (for whey)
- 5 tbsp of lemon juice
- Fresh thyme
- 2 garlic cloves
- Lemon pepper (optional)
- Salt

To the bread:

- 1 egg
- ½ cup liquid marinade
- Wheat flour
- Bread crumbs
- Salt

Steps to Cook

9. Start preparing the buttermilk, put the milk in a container and add the lemon, stir and let it rest for 20 minutes, the milk will thicken. Put the fish fillets on a plate, season with salt and thyme, pour the buttermilk over the fillets, add the thinly sliced garlic, add the lemon pepper or pepper of your choice, cover with plastic wrap and let sit for 30 minutes.

For bread:

1. Place an egg on a plate, mix ½ cup of the marinade liquid, and add a pinch of salt. Pass the fillet in the wheat flour, then in the egg-milk mixture and finish with breadcrumbs. Put in the air fryer for 25 minutes at 400°F. Drizzle a little olive oil in the last 5 minutes in the fryer.

Nutrition Information

- Calories: 221
- Carbohydrates: 8.33g
- Fat: 10.25g
- Protein: 22.52g
- Sugar: 0.76g
- Cholesterol: 85mg

Milanese Steak

Servings: 2
Preparation time: 5 minutes
Cook time: 20 minutes

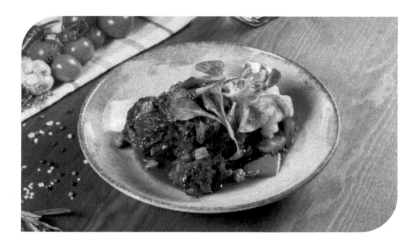

Ingredients

- *Thinly sliced steaks*
- *Egg*
- *Bread crumbs*
- *onion, garlic, salt to taste*

Steps to Cook

1. Season the fillets with the desired seasoning and allow time to absorb the flavor. Then, roll the egg and breadcrumbs into the powder.
2. Finally, place it in the fryer for 20 minutes at 400°F. Turn in half the time.
8. Ready. Enjoy your steak!

Nutrition Information

- Calories: 170
- Carbohydrates: 0g
- Fat: 6g
- Protein: 22g
- Sugar: 0g
- Cholesterol: 240mg

Pork Rind

Servings: 4-6
Preparation time: 10 minutes
Cook time: 45 minutes

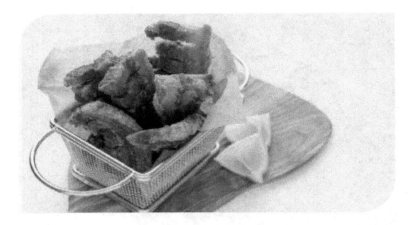

Ingredients

- 2 ¼ pounds pork belly to crunch
- Salt to taste
- 1 pinch of black pepper

Steps to Cook

1. Cut the pork belly into cubes.
2. Then season with salt to taste and a pinch of black pepper.
3. Place in the basket of the Air Fryer.
4. Set the air fryer for 45 minutes at 400°F and stir every 10 minutes.
5. Then simply drain on paper towels and serve.

Nutrition Information

- Calories: 125
- Carbohydrates: 0.5g
- Fat: 9g
- Protein: 16.4g
- Sugar: 0g
- Cholesterol: 32.6mg

Barbecue Picanha

Servings: 4-6
Preparation time: 15 minutes
Cook time: 40 minutes

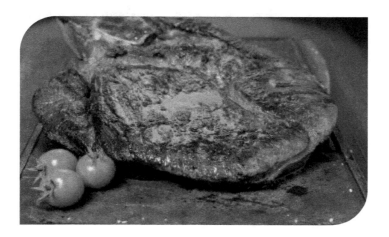

Ingredients

- 2 ¼ lbs of steak
- Coarse salt
- 1 charcoal

Steps to Cook

1. Make small cuts in the thick part of the picanha so that the coarse salt penetrates well. Rub coarse salt on the piece and set aside for a few minutes.
2. Preheat fryer to 400°F. Remove excess salt and place all steak in fryer, fatty side up for 30 minutes.
3. Bring the coal to the fire to make embers. When the meat has time, flip the fat over and place the red hot charcoal in the fryer basket with the fillet.
4. Cook for another 10 minutes and ready!

Nutrition Information

- Calories: 53
- Carbohydrates: 7.3g
- Fat: 2.04g
- Protein: 1.24g
- Sugar: 0.07g
- Cholesterol: 0mg

Greek Barbecue

Servings: 2-4
Preparation time: 5 minutes
Cook time: 35 minutes

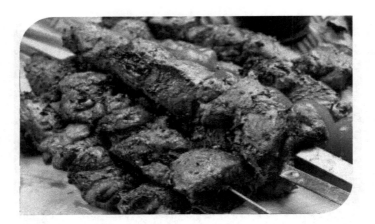

Ingredients

- 1 ¼ lbs of fillet
- ½ red pepper
- ½ green pepper
- 1 onion
- Chile
- Salt

Steps to Cook

1. Cut the fillet into thin fillets. Chop the bell peppers into thin slices and the onion into slices.
2. Place a fillet in the fryer and top with a little of each vegetable. Spice with salt and pepper.
3. Put another fillet on the vegetables and alternate the layers of meat and vegetables until done.
4. Cover the meat with aluminum foil and cook for 25 minutes at 400°F.
5. After that time, remove the foil and bake for another 10 minutes, at the same temperature.

Nutrition Information

- Calories: 145
- Carbohydrates: 1g
- Fat: 5g
- Protein: 21g
- Sugar: 0g
- Cholesterol: 300mg

Barbecue With Skewers

Servings: 4-6
Preparation time: 10 minutes
Cook time: 20 minutes

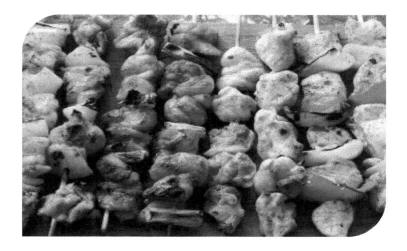

Ingredients

- ½ lb of rump
- ½ lb of chicken fillet
- 3 Tuscan sausages
- Chile
- Salt
- Wooden toothpicks

Steps to Cook

1. Chop the chicken and meat into cubes, and the sausage into slices. Season to taste with pepper and salt.
2. Assemble the skewers, sandwiching the meats.
3. Place the skewers in the fryer basket.
4. Cook for 20 minutes at 400°F.

Nutrition Information

- Calories: 370
- Carbohydrates: 0g
- Fat: 1g
- Protein: 7g
- Sugar: 0g
- Cholesterol: 35mg

Barbecue With Homemade Kafta

Servings: 2-4
Preparation time: 5 minutes
Cook time: 20 minutes

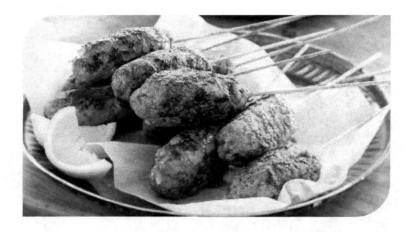

Ingredients

- ½ lb of ground beef
- 1 tbsp of onion cream powder
- 2 cloves of garlic
- ½ lemon;
- Salt.

Steps to Cook

1. Season the garlic and onion mince, add the lemon juice and a little salt. Add the onion cream and mix well. Mold the kafta into barbecue sticks and bring the Air Fryer to 350°F for 10 minutes.
2. Season the ground beef with garlic and onion. Then add a few drops of lemon and a pinch of salt.
3. Add a tablespoon of onion cream to join the kafta. Mold the meat on the barbecue sticks and take it to the fryer for 10 minutes at 350°F.

Nutrition Information

- Calories: 117
- Carbohydrates: 3g
- Fat: 5g
- Protein: 12g
- Sugar: 1g
- Cholesterol: 268mg

Breaded Steak

Servings: 2-4
Preparation time: 5 minutes
Cook time: 20 minutes

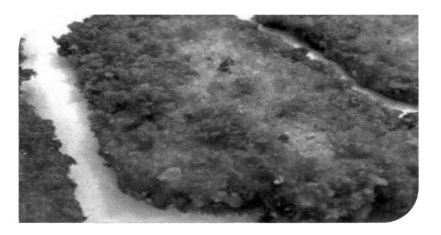

Ingredients

- Thinly sliced steaks
- Egg
- Bread crumbs
- onion
- Garlic
- salt to taste

Steps to Cook

1. Season the fillets with the desired seasoning and allow time to absorb the flavor. Then, roll the egg and breadcrumbs into the powder.
2. Finally, place it in the fryer for 20 minutes at 390°F. Turn in half the time.
3. Ready. Enjoy your steak!

Nutrition Information

- Calories: 301.9
- Carbohydrates: 10.5g
- Fat: 11g
- Protein: 25g
- Sugar: 1g
- Cholesterol: 70mg

Pork Fillet Medallions

Servings: 2-4
Preparation time: 15 mins
Cook time: 25 minutes

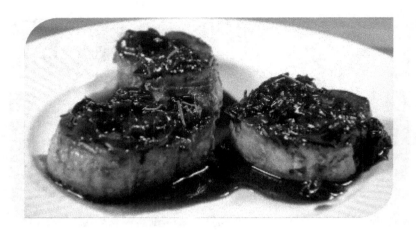

Ingredients

- 4 units of pork fillet with bacon

Steps to Cook

1. Preheat the appliance for 5 minutes, adjusting the temperature to 390°F.
2. Place the medallions in the cooking basket.
3. Set the timer to 25 minutes.
4. Remove and serve while still hot.

Nutrition Information

- Calories: 105.7
- Carbohydrates: 0g
- Fat: 1.7g
- Protein: 22g
- Sugar: 0g
- Cholesterol: 30m

Beef Parmigiana

Servings: 2-4
Preparation time: 5 minutes
Cook time: 11 minutes

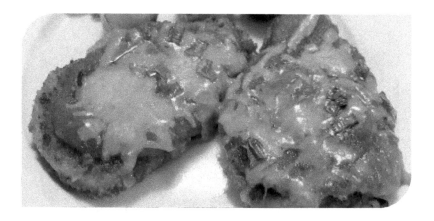

Ingredients

- ½ lb seasoned fillet to taste
- 1 garlic clove, crushed
- 1 oz. of wheat flour
- 1 oz. of breadcrumbs
- 1 egg
- Salt and pepper to taste
- 2 slices of ham
- 2 slices of mozzarella cheese
- 4 tbsp of tomato sauce

Steps to Cook

1. Pass the crushed garlic over the seasoned fillets.
2. Bread the fillets with the flour, egg and breadcrumbs.
3. Place a slice of ham and a slice of cheese on top of the fillets. Add two tablespoons of tomato sauce on top.
4. Preheat the appliance for 5 minutes, adjusting the temperature to 390°F.
5. Place the fillets in the cooking basket.
6. Set the timer to 11 minutes.
7. After 5 minutes, open the tray and carefully rotate the fillets. Close the tray and wait until preparation is complete.
8. Remove and serve hot.

Nutrition Information

- Calories: 236
- Carbohydrates: 31g
- Fat: 4g
- Protein: 17g
- Sugar: 0g
- Cholesterol: 300mg

Meat With Rustic Potatoes

Servings: 4-6
Preparation time: 5 minutes
Cook time: 40 minutes

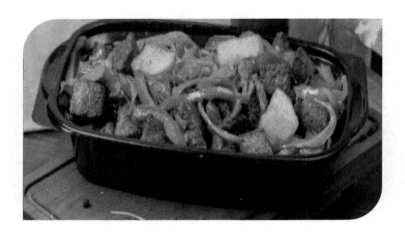

Ingredients

- 2 ¼ lbs of rump
- 4 potatoes
- 1 onion
- 3 garlic cloves
- White wine
- Olive oil
- Salt

Steps to Cook

1. Chop the onion and garlic, place in a bowl with the meat, add the oil and wine and marinate overnight.
2. Preheat the fryer and remove the basket.
3. Place the meat directly in the tub and program to bake at 390°F for 40 minutes.
4. Turn the meat over every 10 minutes, basting it with a little of the marinade liquid. After 20 minutes, add the potatoes in a rustic cut.

Nutrition Information

- Calories: 420
- Carbohydrates: 38g
- Fat: 19g
- Protein: 28g
- Sugar: 5g
- Cholesterol: 45mg

Pumpkin With Beef

Servings: 2
Preparation time: 5 minutes
Cook time: 12 minutes

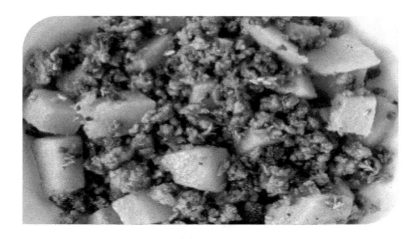

Ingredients

- ½ lb of dried meat;
- ½ lb of pumpkin;
- 1 onion
- Olive oil.

Steps to Cook

1. To remove excess salt, soak the dried meat overnight. After that, cut the meat into thin pieces.
2. Chop the onion well and cut the pumpkin into cubes. Place the 3 ingredients in the Air Fryer basket and drizzle with a drizzle of olive oil.
3. Program to cook for 12 minutes at a temperature of 320°F.

Nutrition Information

- Calories: 135
- Carbohydrates: 8.9g
- Fat: 1.5g
- Protein: 6.9g
- Sugar: 1.2g
- Cholesterol: 30mg

Filet Mignon With Gorgonzola Sauce

Servings: 2-4
Preparation time: 5 minutes
Cook time: 10 minutes

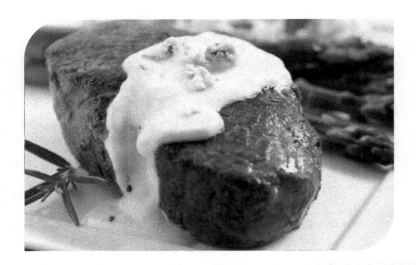

Ingredients

- 4 filet mignon medallions
- 1 cup of curd
- 1 tbsp of gorgonzola cheese
- 2 tbsp of milk
- Black pepper
- Salt

Steps to Cook

1. Season the meat with pepper and salt to taste.
2. Place in the preheated fryer and cook for 10 minutes at 390°F.
3. Meanwhile, prepare the sauce. Take a pan and, over low heat, melt the gorgonzola with the milk. When the medallions are ready, serve covered with the sauce.

Nutrition Information

- Calories: 235.8
- Carbohydrates: 3.36g
- Fat: 19.51g
- Protein: 12g
- Sugar: 0.72g
- Cholesterol: 59.67mg

Meat In Wine Sauce

Servings: 4-6
Preparation time: 10 minutes
Cook time: 8 minutes

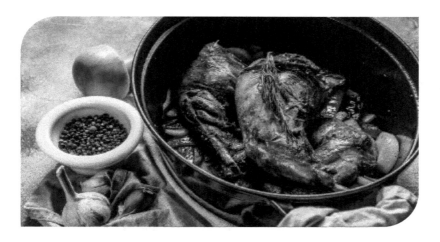

Ingredients

- ½ lb of your favorite minced meat;
- 1 glass of red wine;
- 3 onions cut in half;
- 1 carrot cut into small cubes;
- Meat broth;
- Black pepper;
- Salt.

Steps to Cook

1. Put all ingredients in the fryer basket. Set to bake at 320°F for 30 minutes. If you want a more complete sauce, add a little butter and flour.

Nutrition Information

- Calories: 449.6
- Carbohydrates: 12.4g
- Fat: 29.9g
- Protein: 39.7g
- Sugar: 5.1g
- Cholesterol: 80.5mg

Chapter 6

Seafood Recipes

Fried Manjubinha

Servings: 2-3
Preparation time: 5 minutes
Cook time: 5 minutes

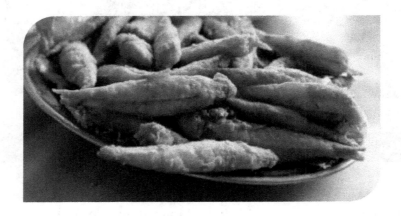

Ingredients

- 1 lb of Manjubinha fish
- 1 tbsp crushed garlic
- 1 tbsp of lemon juice or vinegar
- Salt and black
- 1 egg
- 1 cup of wheat flour
  - 1 cup cornmeal

Steps to Cook

1. Clean and remove the head of each manjubinha. With the clean manjubinhas, place them in a bowl and add the garlic, lemon juice or vinegar, salt and pepper, macerate for at least half an hour. Meanwhile, place the lightly beaten egg in one bowl and in another mix the flour with the cornmeal. Pass each of the manjubinhas in the beaten eggs and then in the flour mixture, sprinkling correctly but without leaving the excess flour. Place half of the manjubinhas carefully in the Air Fryer for 12 to 15 minutes at 400°F and ready.

Nutrition Information

- Calories: 143
- Carbohydrates: 0g
- Fat: 0g
- Protein: 14g
- Sugar: 0g
- Cholesterol: 300mg

Kanikama Stick

Servings: 4
Preparation time: 2 minutes
Cook time: 18 minutes

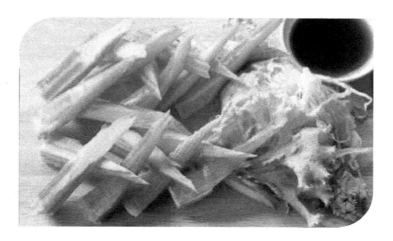

Ingredients

- 5 *Kanikama sticks*

Steps to Cook

1. Remove the packaging from the kanikama and, using a sharp knife, destroy it finely, making fine strips.
2. Place the grated kanikama in the Air Fryer basket and adjust for 15 to 18 minutes at 302°F.
3. Stir several times at least during preparation so that it lasts evenly.

Nutrition Information

- Calories: 121
- Carbohydrates: 17g
- Fat: 0g
- Protein: 11g
- Sugar: 0g
- Cholesterol:30 0mg

Light Fried Fish

Servings: 5
Preparation time: 10 minutes
Cook time: 45 minutes

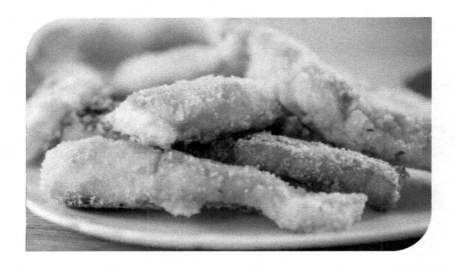

Ingredients

- 5 slices of fish
- 2 tbsp of oat bran or other flour
- 1 lemon
- Salt to taste
- Pepper to taste
- 1 clove garlic, minced

Steps to Cook

1. Season the fish with lemon juice, garlic, pepper and salt.
2. Pass the slices into the bran.
3. Put in the air fryer for 20 to 25 minutes at 350°F.

Nutrition Information

- Calories: 190
- Carbohydrates: 24g
- Fat: 6g
- Protein: 11g
- Sugar: 3g
- Cholesterol: 15mg

SHRIMP

Servings: 4
Preparation time: 5 minutes
Cook time: 20 minutes

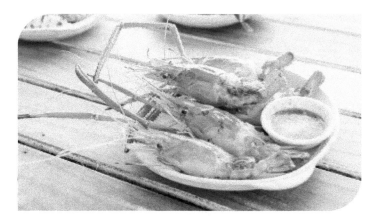

Ingredients

- 2 ¼ lbs of clean shrimp
- Fresh basil
- Leek
- thyme
- Garlic
- olive oil to taste

Steps to Cook

1. Season the prawns and leave them in a bowl for at least 15 minutes.
2. Place in fryer for 20 minutes at 390°F.
3. Ready! Just enjoy the fat-free shrimp!

Nutrition Information

- Calories: 101
- Carbohydrates: 1.3g
- Fat: 1.4g
- Protein: 19g
- Sugar: 0g
- Cholesterol: 179mg

Cod

Servings: 2-4
Preparation time: 10 minutes
Cook time: 35 minutes

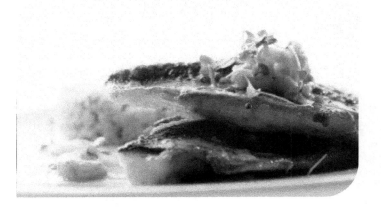

Ingredients

- 1 pound of cod
- 1 lb potato ball
- 1 ½ oz olive
- Salt
- black pepper
- Pepper
- Cherry tomato
- Garlic
- Onion
- Olive oil to taste.

Steps to Cook

1. Add the cod to desalinate. Meanwhile, wash the potatoes, pat dry, place them on the fryer pan, sprinkle with salt and oil, and turn on the 390°F for 15 minutes.
2. Then add the cod and add the spices to taste. Put another 20 minutes at 390°F and you're done. Your cod will be ready.

Nutrition Information

- Calories: 90
- Carbohydrates: 0g
- Fat: 1g
- Protein: 20g
- Sugar: 0g
- Cholesterol: 41mg

Breaded Fillet Of Hake

Servings: 2
Preparation time: 5 minutes
Cook time: 13 minutes

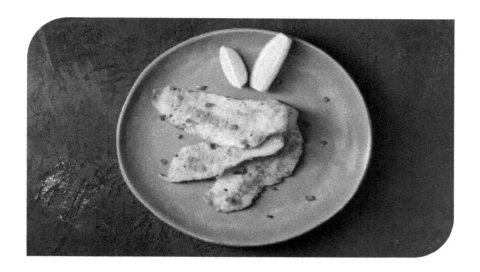

Ingredients

- 1 pound fillet of hake
- 3 garlic cloves, crushed
- Salt and pepper to taste
- 1/3 cup wheat flour
- 2 lightly beaten eggs
- 2 cups panko or toasted breadcrumbs

Steps to Cook

1. Season the fish fillets with garlic, salt and pepper. Pass the fish through wheat flour, egg and finally panko. Remove the excess panko and place it in the Air Fryer basket, already preheated to 400°F for 3 minutes. Bake for about 10 minutes at 400°F, or until the cone is golden. Remove and serve with lemon wedges and tartar sauce.

Nutrition Information

- Calories: 193
- Carbohydrates: 7g
- Fat: 6g
- Protein: 25g
- Sugar: 0g
- Cholesterol: 300mg

Fish Bait

Servings: 4-6
Preparation time: 5 minutes
Cook time: 15 minutes

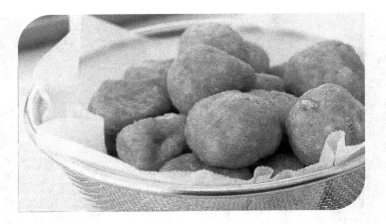

Ingredients

- ½ lb of fish fillet
- 2 eggs
- ½ lb of breadcrumbs
- ½ lb of wheat flour
- 1 lemon
- salt to taste

Steps to Cook

1. First cut the fillet into strips
2. Place in a container and season with salt and lemon.
3. Mix well
4. Dip the strips one by one in the wheat flour, eggs and breadcrumbs
5. Put the baits in the fryer
6. Set the timer for 8 minutes at 390°F.
7. After that time it is ready

Nutrition Information

- Calories: 218
- Carbohydrates: 0g
- Fat: 4.5g
- Protein: 44g
- Sugar: 0g
- Cholesterol: 97mg

Tilapia Fillet

Servings: 4
Preparation time: 5 minutes
Cook time: 10 minutes

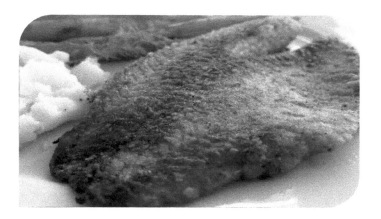

Ingredients

- 1 lb of tilapia fillet
- 1 lemon
- Salt to taste
- Dehydrated thyme

Steps to Cook

1. Season the fillet with salt and lemon.
2. Heat the pan for two minutes over medium heat.
3. Place the open fillets in the pan and sprinkle the thyme on top.
4. Drizzle with a drizzle of olive oil.
5. Put in the air fryer for 3 minutes at $320°F$ to brown and change in the other side.

Nutrition Information

- Calories: 218
- Carbohydrates: 0g
- Fat: 4.5g
- Protein: 44g
- Sugar: 0g
- Cholesterol: 97mg

Tilapia on Papillot

Servings: 2
Preparation time: 5 minutes
Cook time: 10 minutes

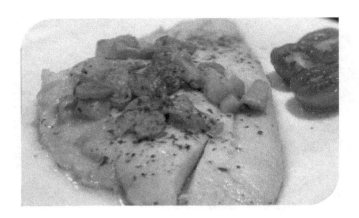

Ingredients

- 2 tilapia fillets
- 1 small sweet potato
- 1 tomato cut into slices
- Lemon to taste
- Salt to taste
- Black pepper to taste
- Olive oil to taste
- 2 pieces of aluminum foil

Steps to Cook

1. Season the fillets with lemon, salt and pepper. Marinate and meanwhile wash the tomatoes and potatoes and cut them into slices.
2. Place the potato slices on the foil and season the potato with salt.
3. Place the seasoned fillets on the potato layer, the tomato slices on the fish and drizzle with olive oil.
4. Close the foil bags.
9. Take to the fryer to 390°F for 25-30 minutes.

Nutrition Information

- Calories: 218
- Carbohydrates: 0g
- Fat: 4.5g
- Protein: 44g
- Sugar: 0g
- Cholesterol: 97mg

Coconut Breaded Shrimp

Servings: 4
Preparation time: 5 minutes
Cook time: 7 minutes

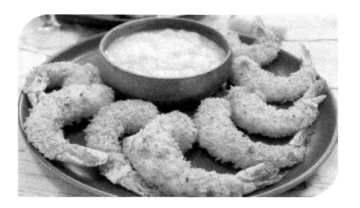

Ingredients

- ½ lb shrimp
- 1 ½ oz. of breadcrumbs
- 1 ½ oz. of grated coconut
- 1 ½ oz. of panko
- Salt and pepper to taste
- 1 lemon
- 1 egg

Steps to Cook

1. Season the prawns with salt, pepper and lemon.
2. In a shallow dish, place the flour.
3. Chop the parsley and mix in a bowl with the coconut, panko and breadcrumbs.
4. Bread the prawns in the flour and egg, and the flour mixture.
5. Preheat the appliance for 5 minutes, adjusting the temperature to 390°F.
6. Place the prawns in the cooking basket leaving a small space among them.
7. Set the timer to 7 minutes.
8. Remove and serve hot.

Nutrition Information

- Calories: 310
- Carbohydrates: 31g
- Fat: 16g
- Protein: 9g
- Sugar: 10g
- Cholesterol: 50mg

Salmon With Orange Sauce

Servings: 2
Preparation time: 5 minutes
Cook time: 5 minutes

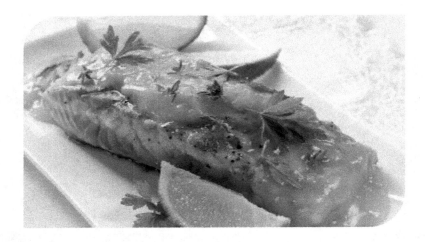

Ingredients

- ½ lb salmon fillet
- ½ cup of orange juice
- 1 tbsp cornstarch
- Salt and black pepper to taste.

Steps to Cook

1. Season the salmon with salt and pepper, according to your preference
2. Preheat the air fryer for 5 minutes, adjusting the temperature to 390°F.
3. Place the salmon in the cooking basket.
4. Set the timer to 5 minutes.
5. In a saucepan, place the orange juice, salt, pepper and cornstarch.
6. Stir with the help of a fouet and boil for 2 minutes. Reserve.
7. Remove the salmon from the cooking basket.
8. On a plate, place the salmon and orange sauce on top. Serve it hot.

Nutrition Information

- Calories: 602
- Carbohydrates: 35g
- Fat: 28g
- Protein: 51g
- Sugar: 30g
- Cholesterol: 143mg

Cod With Breadcrumbs

Servings: 4-6
Preparation time: 5 minutes
Cook time: 25 minutes

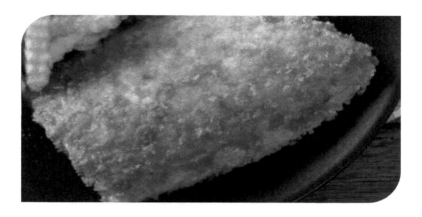

Ingredients

- 2 large onions, chopped
- 1 lb of ripe tomatoes
- 1 cup chopped parsley
- 3 ½ oz. green olives
- 1 cup black raisins
- 3 ½ oz. chopped walnuts
- ½ cup Parmesan cheese
- 2 packages bread crumbled
- Salt to taste
- 1 cup olive oil
- 2 ½ lb of shredded cod, soaked and boiled
- 6 ripe tomatoes, cut into 0.5 cm thick slices

Steps to Cook

1. In a bowl, mix together the onion, diced tomatoes, parsley, olives, raisins, walnuts, and Parmesan.
2. Add the crumbled bread and check the seasoning.
3. If necessary, add salt.
4. Add a little olive oil to get very moist flour.
5. In a refractory form, mix layers of breadcrumbs, cod, and tomato slices until all ingredients are finished.
6. Drizzle with remaining oil and place in the air fryer preheated at 390°F for 25 minutes or until golden.

Nutrition Information

- Calories: 156
- Carbohydrates: 16.4g
- Fat: 0.2g
- Protein: 16.6g
- Sugar: 1.9g
- Cholesterol: 0mg

Fried Squid

Servings: 2-4
Preparation time: 5 minutes
Cook time: 5 minutes

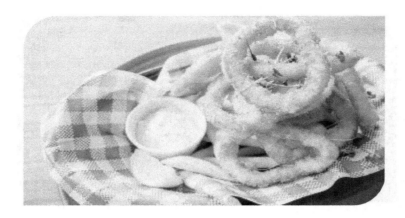

Ingredients

- ½ lb squid rings
- 1 medium onion unit
- 1 tablespoon of olive oil
- white pepper to taste
- 1 bay leaf

Steps to Cook

1. Season the squid with salt, garlic, pepper, and bay leaf. Let marinate for a while.
2. Cut the onion into slices and place in the Air Fryer along with the squid and a tablespoon of oil and let it brown for 5 minutes at 320°F.

Nutrition Information

- Calories: 148
- Carbohydrates: 6.6g
- Fat: 6.4g
- Protein: 15.2g
- Sugar: 0g
- Cholesterol: 221mg

Fish With Vegetables

Servings: 1
Preparation time: 5 minutes
Cook time: 20-25 minutes

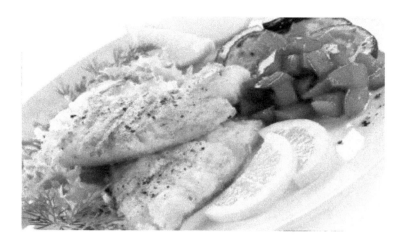

Ingredients

- 2 pieces of aluminum foil
- 2 fish fillets (hake, tilapia, sole)
- 2 medium potatoes, thinly sliced
- 1 medium tomato, thinly sliced
- 2 tbsp sliced olives
- Lemon to taste
- Salt to taste
- Black pepper to taste
- Olive oil to taste

Steps to Cook

1. Season the fish with lemon, salt and pepper.
2. Place the potato slices on the foil.
3. Season the potato with salt.
4. Lay the seasoned fish on top of the potato layer.
5. Place the tomato slices on the fish layer.
6. Add the olives
7. Drizzle with olive oil.
8. Close the aluminum foil.
9. Take to the Air fryer at 390°F for 20-25 minutes.

Nutrition Information

- Calories: 196.7
- Carbohydrates: 5.9g
- Fat: 8.6g
- Protein: 24.2g
- Sugar: 2.2g
- Cholesterol: 55.2mg

Sardine Pizza

Servings: 2-4
Preparation time: 5 minutes
Cook time: 30 minutes

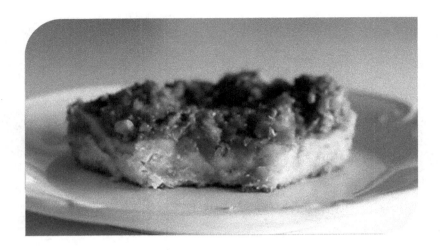

Ingredients

- 1 ½ cups warm water
- 1 tsp salt
- 1 tbsp of low sugar
- 5 tbsp of oil
- 2 eggs
- 1 sachet of yeast for bread

Sauce:

- 1 medium onion, chopped
- 1 chopped tomato
- 1 can of sardine
- 1 sachet of tomato extract

Steps to Cook

1. Mix yeast, water, sugar, salt and oil.
2. Place the whole eggs and little by little the flour.
3. Beat the dough well, almost cake texture, a little firmer
4. Place in a large rectangular shape, greased and floured, and let it grow for 30 minutes.
5. Put in the air fryer at 350°F for about 10 minutes, add sauce and bake for another 20 minutes.
6. To make the sauce, fry the onion and add the tomato. Fry the sardines together.
7. Put the sauce, salt, boil a little and turn off. You can add black pepper!

Nutrition Information

- Calories: 125
- Carbohydrates: 0g
- Fat: 7g
- Protein: 14.8g
- Sugar: 3g
- Cholesterol: 0mg

Cod With Capers

Servings: 3
Preparation time: 5 minutes
Cook time: 15 minutes

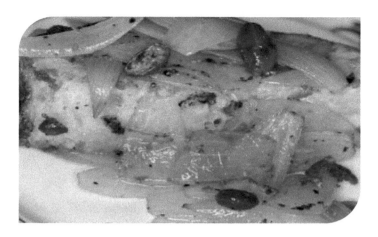

Ingredients

- 2 ½ desalted cod, sliced
- 8 tbsp of olive oil
- 2 large onions
- ½ cup of capers
- 1 clove garlic

Steps to Cook

1. Preheat the air fryer at 350°F and add the pieces of cod and roast for 15 minutes or until golden brown.
2. When they are golden brown, rotate them with tweezers or a spatula, being very careful not to disassemble the slices.
3. Cut the onions into petals and drain the capers.
4. Remove the pieces from the pan and set aside in a warm place to keep them warm.
5. In a pan add oil, onion, capers, lemon and vinegar. Let it brown well until the onions are transparent. Get salt and pepper.
6. Serve by placing the sauce over the cod.

Nutrition Information

- Calories: 226
- Carbohydrates: 6.9g
- Fat: 2.7g
- Protein: 40.6g
- Sugar: 2.4g
- Cholesterol: 99.1m

Tilapia With Mushrooms And Paprika

Servings: 1-2
Preparation time: 5 minutes
Cook time: 20 minutes

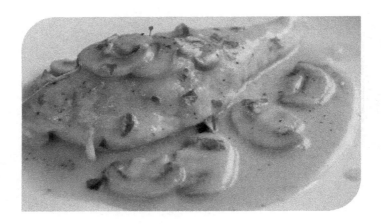

Ingredients

- 1 lb of tilapia fillet
- ½ lb of fresh mushroom
- to taste cherry tomatoes
- 1/3 cup of white wine
- 1 tbsp of smoked paprika
- Parsley and chives to taste
- Salt and pepper to taste

Steps to Cook

1. In a baking dish, distribute the fillets and season with salt and pepper.
2. Disinfect and cut mushrooms and tomatoes. Distribute over the fish.
3. Add the white wine and sprinkle the paprika over the fillets.
4. Put in the air fryer for about 20 minutes at 350°F.
5. After roasting, add the parsley and chives. Serve with rice or potatoes, It's great!

Nutrition Information

- Calories: 184.3
- Carbohydrates: 2.7g
- Fat: 10.9g
- Protein: 21.7g
- Sugar: 0.5g
- Cholesterol: 0mg

Tilapia With Sweet Potatoes

Servings: 1
Preparation time: 5 minutes
Cook time: 40 minutes

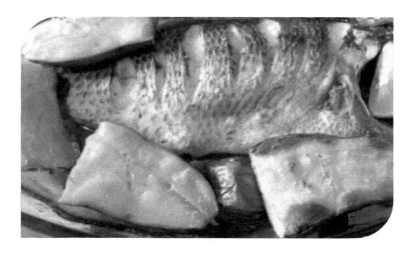

Ingredients

- 1 tilapia
- 2 sweet potatoes
- 2 onion
- 2 cloves of garlic
- 1 basil branch
- to taste pepper and salt
- 1 lemon

Steps to Cook

1. Season the tilapia with salt and lemon and put the crushed garlic and pepper and the basil inside the tilapia and place them in the marinex and reserve.
2. Cut the potato into large pieces and pre-cook. Then place it next to the tilapia.
3. Cut the onion into a large piece and place it around the tilapia, take it to a preheated air fryer at 350^0F until it begins to brown, about 40 minutes.

Nutrition Information

- Calories: 290
- Carbohydrates: 31g
- Fat: 3.5g
- Protein: 37g
- Sugar: 10g
- Cholesterol: 65mg

Chapter 7

Air Fryer Vegetables Recipes

Lentil Dumpling

Servings: 40-45
Preparation time: 20 minutes
Cook time: 15-20 minutes

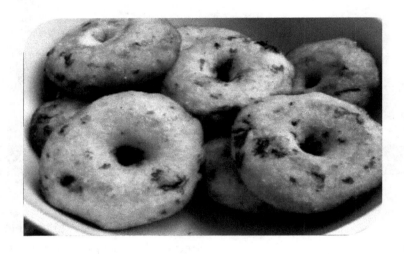

Ingredients

- 1 cup dried lentils
- 3 cups of water
- ½ tbsp of salt
- 1 Cup of wheat for kibbeh
- 1 cup chopped vegetables
- ½ grated or shredded onion
- 1 tbsp crushed garlic
- 1 tbsp of olive oil
- ½ cup green aroma
  - 1 tbsp of wheat flour

Steps to Cook

1. In a pressure cooker, place the lentils, water and salt, cover and cook for 20 minutes.
2. Meanwhile, in another skillet, sauté the deli, greens, or vegetables of your choice along with the onion, garlic, and olive oil.
3. As soon as the lentils are ready, pour them into a bowl, with water and everything, and add the stir fry you made, the wheat for kebab, the green aroma and the wheat flour.
4. Mix everything well and let cool.
5. After the dough is cold, shape the meatballs and place them on a baking sheet greased with oil, and then put them in the freezer to freeze.
6. When ready, place as many cookies as you can in the Air Fryer's basket, without piling up too much, and set

the Air Fryer for 15-20 minutes at 400°F, until they begin to brown slightly.

Nutrition Information

- Calories: 93
- Carbohydrates: 13g
- Fat: 3g

- Protein: 4g
- Sugar: 0g
- Cholesterol: 300mg

Risotto Balls

Servings: 4
Preparation time: 60 minutes
Cook time: 13 minutes

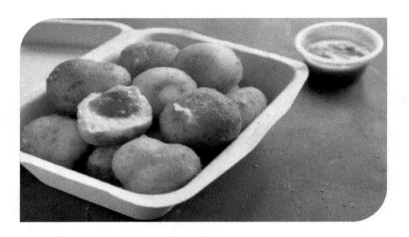

Ingredients

- Risotto
- Wheat flour
- Egg white
- Toasted breadcrumbs

Steps to Cook

1. You will need the risotto from the day before first, preferably frozen, you can leave the risotto.
2. With the frozen risotto make balls, then roll these balls in the wheat flour, then the egg whites and finally the toasted breadcrumbs, remember not to leave the excess flour, you just want a thin and crispy cone and the moist risotto for inside.
3. Take the cookies to freeze and after freezing put them in the Air Fryer basket and prepare for 13 minutes at 400°F.

Nutrition Information

- Calories: 47
- Carbohydrates: 5.4g
- Fat: 2g
- Protein: 1.7g
- Sugar: 0.2g
- Cholesterol: 9.7mg

Fried Soybeans

Servings: 4
Preparation time: 30 minutes
Cook time: 15 minutes

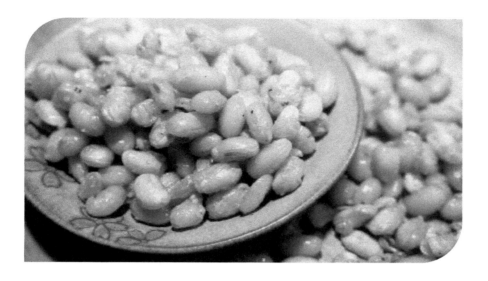

Ingredients

- 1 cup raw soybeans
- ½ tsp of salt for a mild flavor or 1 teaspoon of salt for more snacks

Steps to Cook

1. Place soybeans in a bowl and cover with about 5 cups of water, soak overnight, at least 12 hours.
2. The next day the soy will be hydrated and softer, discard this water and add another, rub and squeeze the soybeans between your hands in the water, gently to split them in half and the shells can be released, they will float on the beans, remove all shells, drain and follow well. Mix the salt in the soy. If your basket has holes, line the bottom with a piece of aluminum foil and pour the soy into the basket.
3. Put in the Air Fryer for 20 to 30 minutes at 400°F, shaking the basket every 5 minutes.

Nutrition Information

- Calories: 350
- Carbohydrates: 40g
- Fat: 5g
- Protein: 6g
- Sugar: 5g
- Cholesterol: 300mg

Brazilian Pine Nuts

Servings: 2-4
Preparation time: 5 minutes
Cook time: 10 minutes

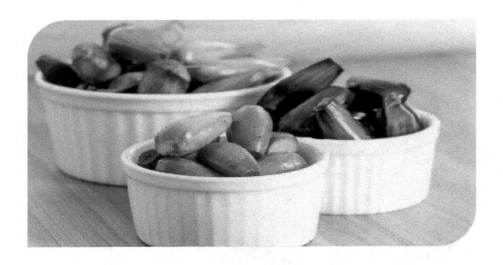

Ingredients

- ½ lb pine nuts

Steps to Cook

1. Thoroughly wash pine nuts in water, and then dry thoroughly.
2. Using a good pair of scissors, cut the ends of each pine nuts.
3. If you don't have good scissors, use a sharp knife.
4. Now place the pine nuts in the Air Fryer basket, already preheated, and program for 10 minutes at 400°F, stirring the basket in half the time.
5. After the time, the pine nuts are ready.

Nutrition Information

- Calories: 67
- Carbohydrates: 15.34g
- Fat: 0.2g
- Protein: 1.04g
- Sugar: 0.06g
- Cholesterol: 0mg

Breadcrumbs With Dried Fruit

Servings: 2
Preparation time: 10 minutes
Cook time: 40 minutes

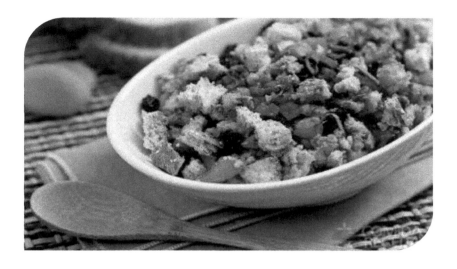

Ingredients

- 2 slices of whole wheat bread
- 1 tbsp chopped chives
- ¼ cup raisins
- ¼ cup small diced apricots
- ½ orange juice
- Syrian pepper to taste

Steps to Cook

1. Cut the loaves into very small pieces or tear them by hand.
2. On a baking sheet, place the crumbled breads, raisins, apricots, orange juice, and pepper.
3. Put the pan in the air fryer for 30 minutes or until the flour is slightly crisp at 400°F.
4. Add the chives and serve.

Nutrition Information

- Calories: 140
- Carbohydrates: 15g
- Fat: 9g
- Protein: 4g
- Sugar: 11g
- Cholesterol: 0mg

Eggplant Paste

Servings: 2
Preparation time: 5 minutes
Cook time: 15 minutes

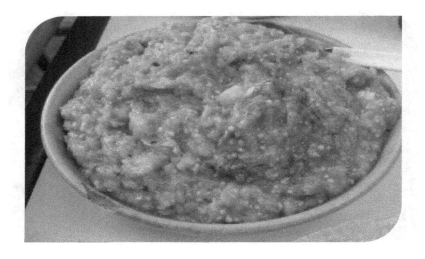

Ingredients

- 2 aubergines
- 1 clove garlic
- 1 tbsp of lemon juice
- 2 tbsp tahini
- 2 tbsp of olive oil
- Salt, paprika and pepper to taste.

Steps to Cook

1. Wash the eggplants well and pat dry.
2. Using a knife, drill a few holes and place them in the fryer for 15 minutes at 400°F.
3. Once done, remove the eggplants from the machine and place them on a plate.
4. Cut them in half and, with the help of a spoon, remove all the pulp.
5. Place the eggplant pulp and the other ingredients in a blender or food processor, until it turns into a paste.
6. Transfer the pasta to another container and let it cool or put it in the refrigerator to serve ice cream.
7. When serving, drizzle with a pinch of olive oil and sprinkle with paprika, pepper, and chives on top.

Nutrition Information

- Calories: 30
- Carbohydrates: 2g
- Fat: 2g
- Protein: 1g
- Sugar: 0g
- Cholesterol: 0mg

Cereal Bar

Servings: 4-6
Preparation time: 10 minutes
Cook time: 20 minutes

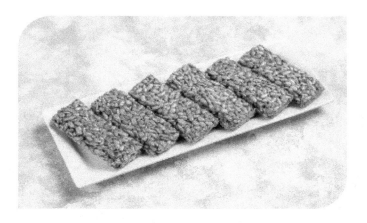

Ingredients

- 3 tbsp margarine
- ½ cup of water
- 1 tbsp of shallow cornstarch
- 2 tbsp of brown sugar
- 5 tbsp of granola
- 5 tbsp Nestlé flakes

Steps to Cook

1. In a saucepan, heat the margarine, water, corn, and sugar.
2. Stir all the time until it thickens and turns off. Put the rest of the ingredients on a plate and pour the mixture over the pan while it is still hot, mix for about 3 minutes.
3. Place the mixture on a baking sheet, leaving a layer 1 cm high. When done, carefully remove and let it warm up; cut into bars and let cool before consuming.
4. In Air Fryer, program for 20 minutes at 320^0F.

Nutrition Information

- Calories: 140
- Carbohydrates: 26g
- Fat: 3g
- Protein: 2g
- Sugar: 13g
- Cholesterol: 0mg

Fried Capeletti

Servings: 10
Preparation time: 5 minutes
Cook time: 30 minutes

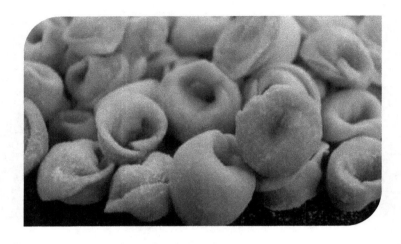

Ingredients

- 2 ¼ lb of homemade Capeletti

Steps to Cook

1. Preheat the air fryer at 400°F for a few minutes. Gradually add the capeletti.
2. Let it fry for 30 minutes or until golden brown (without letting it burn).
3. Remove and place in a container.
4. If necessary, sprinkle a little salt on top and you're done.
5. A good aperitif for the weekend.

Nutrition Information

- Calories: 478
- Carbohydrates: 56g
- Fat: 12g
- Protein: 25g
- Sugar: 0g
- Cholesterol: 300mg

Caponata With Aubergines And Zucchini

Servings: 2-4
Preparation time: 5 minutes
Cook time: 19 minutes

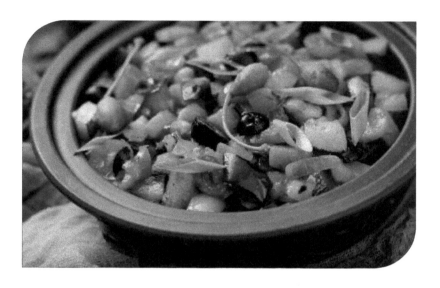

Ingredients

- 1 medium eggplant
- 2 small Italian zucchini
- 1 medium onion
- Salt, black pepper, parsley and chives to taste.
- If you want you can add a little olive oil.
- Salt and black pepper to taste.

Steps to Cook

1. Preheat the air fryer for about 4 minutes, then place the diced eggplant, zucchini, and onion (do not cut into thin slices as they will burn), in a container that can fit inside the Air Fryer or in the basket that comes with nonstick marmitex or other that can enter the oven, mix the ingredients with a little salt, black pepper, oregano and olive oil, bake in the Air Fryer for 15 minutes at 400°F, stir half the time. Check if you like it, if not, put a few more minutes. Put parsley and chives when ready.

Nutrition Information

- Calories: 55
- Carbohydrates: 2g
- Fat: 4.5g
- Protein: 2g
- Sugar: 0g
- Cholesterol: 0mg

Spinach Balls

Servings: 2-4
Preparation time: 2 minutes
Cook time: 20 minutes

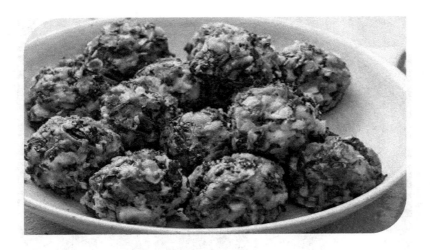

Ingredients

- 1 package of cooked spinach
- 1 cup of grated carrot
- 1 cup all-purpose flour
- 2 eggs
- 1 tsp of baking powder
- ½ chopped onion
- Parsley to taste
- Salt and pepper

Steps to Cook

1. To cook spinach it is easy: put a pan of water on the fire, when it boils put the spinach leaves. Leave for about 2 minutes and remove. Put in a strainer and remove as much water as possible, leaving it very dry. After it is dry, it is good to cut the leaves a little to make it smaller for the cookie
2. Add all ingredients and season with salt and pepper to taste
3. Bring to the air fryer at 350°F for 20 minutes, turning the cookies over half the time.

Nutrition Information

- Calories: 37.1
- Carbohydrates: 2.1g
- Fat: 2.4g
- Protein: 2.3g
- Sugar: 0.2g
- Cholesterol: 28.1mg

Quick Vegetable Pie

Servings: 4
Preparation time: 5 minutes
Cook time: 5 minutes

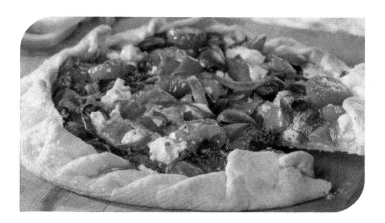

Ingredients

- 6 tbsp mix ready for tapioca MISTER TAP
- 2 eggs
- Vegetables: Tomatoes, selected vegetables, corn, and chopped potatoes.
- Salt to taste
- 1 tbsp of light cheese

Steps to Cook

1. Mix it all up and put it in the air fryer!
2. Set the time to 5 minutes at 350°F.

Nutrition Information

- Calories: 194
- Carbohydrates: 32g
- Fat: 5g
- Protein: 4g
- Sugar: 0g
- Cholesterol: 0mg

Vegetables With Herbs

Servings: 2-4
Preparation time: 5 minutes
Cook time: 15 minutes

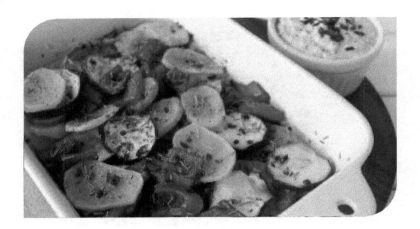

Ingredients

- 1 large carrot, sliced
- 3 large potatoes cut into thick slices
- salt to taste
- lemon pepper to taste
- hot paprika to taste
- herbs to taste
- 1 tbsp of olive oil

Steps to Cook

1. Cut the carrot and potato into slices of 1 cm each.
2. Soak them in a bowl of water for 10 minutes.
3. Then remove all the water, add the spices and oil and mix well. Place the vegetables in the Air Fryer basket and adjust for 15 minutes at 400°F. Half the time, turn the vegetables over to cook evenly. After that time, remove and serve.

Nutrition Information

- Calories: 22
- Carbohydrates: 2.7g
- Fat: 0.6g
- Protein: 3.2g
- Sugar: 0g
- Cholesterol: 0mg

Assorted Vegetables

Servings: 4-6
Preparation time: 10 minutes
Cook time: 20 minutes

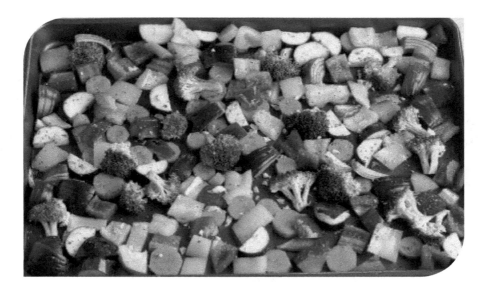

Ingredients

- ½ beet
- 4 pods
- ¼ red pepper
- ¼ yellow pepper
- 1 zucchini
- 15 cherry tomatoes
- ½ carrot
- 1 onion

Steps to Cook

1. Preheat your air fryer for 5 minutes at 400°F.
2. Cut the vegetables into small cubes to facilitate cooking. Put the vegetables in a bowl of water and then rinse. Put all the vegetables in the preheated fryer and cook for 6 minutes at 400°F or until al dente. Season to try and serve.

Nutrition Information

- Calories: 22
- Carbohydrates: 2.7g
- Fat: 0.6g
- Protein: 3.2g
- Sugar: 0g
- Cholesterol: 0mg

5 Roasted Vegetables

Servings: 2-4
Preparation time: 5 minutes
Cook time: 7 minutes

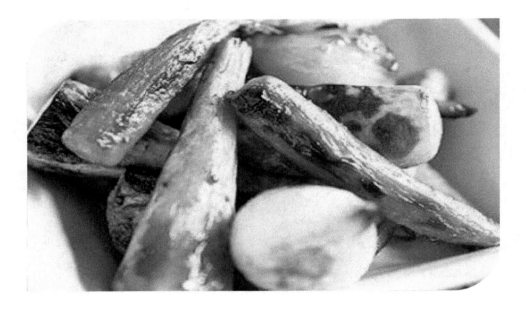

Ingredients

- 1 *zucchini*
- 1 *sweet potato*
- 1 *carrot*
- 1 *onion*
- 1 *tomato*

Steps to Cook

1. Cut the potato, carrot and zucchini into toothpicks. Chop the onion and tomato and mix with the sticks. Add olive oil just to slightly moisten the vegetables.
2. Place in the basket of the Air Fryer and set for 7 minutes at 400°F.
3. Season with salt and pepper and serve. Vegetables are crispy and delicious.

Nutrition Information

- Calories: 22
- Carbohydrates: 2.7g
- Fat: 0.6g
- Protein: 3.2g
- Sugar: 0g
- Cholesterol: 0mg

Roasted Zucchini

Servings: 2-4
Preparation time: 5 minutes
Cook time: 15 minutes

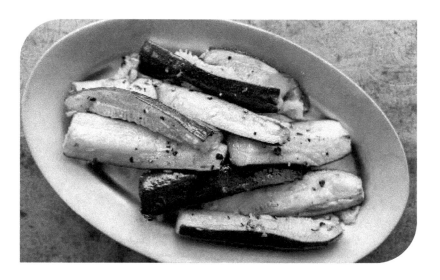

Ingredients

- 1 zucchini cut into sticks
- 2 tbsp of grated cheese
- 1 tbsp of sesame oil
- salt to taste
- Black pepper to taste

Steps to Cook

1. Wash the zucchini under running water. Cut into 3 or 4 slices 1 cm wide. Cut these slices into long sticks, also 1 cm wide. Cut the sticks into 3 parts.
2. Season with black pepper salt to taste. Distribute the sesame oil and the grated cheese on the sticks, wrapping well. Place in the basket and set for 15 minutes at 400°F. Serve!

Nutrition Information

- Calories: 5
- Carbohydrates: 1g
- Fat: 0g
- Protein: 0g
- Sugar: 0.5g
- Cholesterol: 0mg

Carrot Roasted

Servings: 2-4
Preparation time: 5 minutes
Cook time: 20 minutes

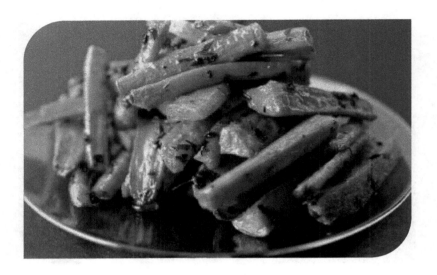

Ingredients

- 3 medium carrots
- 1 tbsp of honey
- 1 tbsp of olive oil
- 1 tbsp of balsamic vinegar
- ½ tsp salt
- 1 pinch of nutmeg
- paprika to taste
- herbs to taste

Steps to Cook

1. Wash the carrots, peel and remove the tips.
2. Then cut into 1 cm sticks. Mix with spices, oil, honey and aceto, mixing well.
3. Place in the fryer basket without oil and set for 20 minutes at 350°F.
4. Half the time, remove and mix to brown evenly. Serve!

Nutrition Information

- Calories: 109
- Carbohydrates: 14g
- Fat: 5.8g
- Protein: 1.4g
- Sugar: 7g
- Cholesterol: 0m

Vegetables With Coconut Oil

Servings: 1-2
Preparation time: 5 minutes
Cook time: 15 minutes

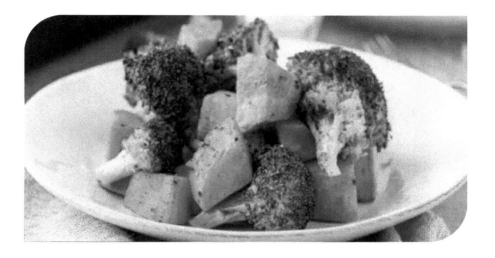

Ingredients

- ½ zucchini, chopped;
- 1 chopped chayote;
- ½ cauliflower, chopped;
- ½ chopped broccoli;
- 1 carrot, chopped;
- Coconut oil to moisten.

Steps to Cook

1. Cut the vegetables into small cubes or smaller pieces.
2. Season with salt, parsley, black pepper, and other spices you like and like.
3. Add a little coconut oil to moisten the vegetables.
4. Distribute in the Air Fryer basket and set for 15 minutes at 400°F.

Nutrition Information

- Calories: 40
- Carbohydrates: 0g
- Fat: 4.5g
- Protein: 0g
- Sugar: 0g
- Cholesterol: 0mg

Roasted Eggplant

Servings: 2-4
Preparation time: 5 minutes
Cook time: 15 minutes

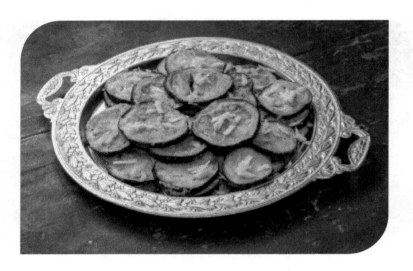

Ingredients

- 2 chopped aubergines
- 2 tbsp of olive oil
- salt to taste;
- black pepper to taste;
- herbs to taste

Steps to Cook

1. Wash the eggplants well and cut them into small pieces. They can be cubes, the smaller, and the easier to cook in the Air Fryer.
2. Season with salt, pepper, and herbs. Put the oil and spread it well on the pieces.
3. Place in the basket and set for 15 minutes at 350^0F. Withdraw and serve!

Nutrition Information

- Calories: 49.6
- Carbohydrates: 4.9g
- Fat: 1.4g
- Protein: 1.6g
- Sugar: 0g
- Cholesterol: 0mg

Fried Chickpeas

Servings: 2-4
Preparation time: 5 minutes
Cook time: 20 minutes

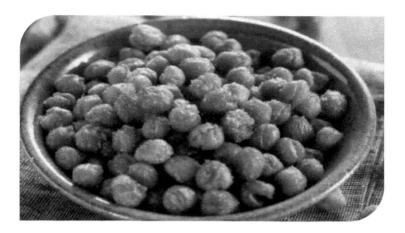

Ingredients

- Cooked chickpeas
- Olive oil
- Black pepper
- Peppers

Steps to Cook

1. Cook the chickpeas for 5 minutes after pressing.
2. Drain the chickpeas immediately.
3. Drain the broth and, in the fryer basket, mix the spices well. Bake at 350°F for 20 minutes.
4. It is super crispy.

Nutrition Information

- Calories: 375
- Carbohydrates: 27g
- Fat: 24g
- Protein: 13g
- Sugar: 2g
- Cholesterol: 276mg

Eggplant lasagna

Servings: 2-4
Preparation time: 5 minutes
Cook time: 35 minutes

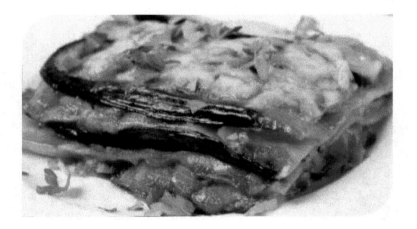

Ingredients

- 3 mini eggplants
- 2 cups of tomato sauce
- cauliflower and broccoli to taste
- 1 lb of mozzarella

Steps to Cook

1. Cut the eggplants vertically; place them in the Air fryer for 15 minutes at 390°F. Remove and start assembling in layers in a heat resistant refractory that fits in your deep fryer, first put the sauce on and then alternate layers of eggplant, sauce, vegetables and cheese until done. Place in the Air fryer for 20 minutes at 320°F and serve.

Nutrition Information

- Calories: 264.2
- Carbohydrates: 26.7g
- Fat: 9.4g
- Protein: 20.3g
- Sugar: 2.4g
- Cholesterol: 25mg

Vegetable Mix

Servings: 2-4
Preparation time: 5 minutes
Cook time: 7 minutes

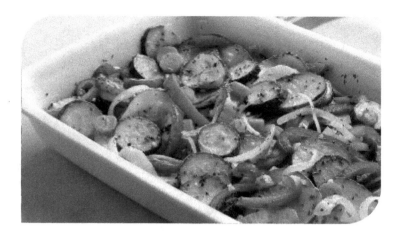

Ingredients

- 1 peeled potato
- 1 zucchini
- 1 carrot
- 1 tomato
- 1 onion
- 1 red pepper
- salt to taste
- a pinch of olive oil

Steps to Cook

1. Cut the potato, carrot and zucchini into toothpicks
2. Chop the tomato and onion into cubes
3. Mix all
4. Drizzle with olive oil, season with salt
5. Take Air Fryer for 7 minutes at 390°F. Serve!

Nutrition Information

- Calories: 45
- Carbohydrates: 9.7g
- Fat: 0.5g
- Protein: 2.4 g
- Sugar: 3.7g
- Cholesterol: 0mg

Eggplant Sticks

Servings: 2-4
Preparation time: 5 minutes
Cook time: 8 minutes

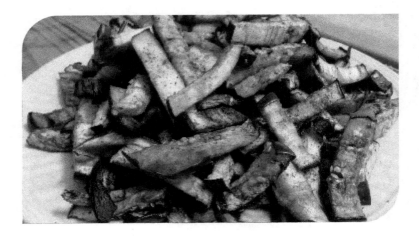

Ingredients

- 1 eggplant cut into sticks
- 2 tbsp of grated cheese
- 1 tbsp of olive oil
- Salt and black pepper to taste.

Steps to Cook

1. Wash 1 medium eggplant under running water. Keep the peel and cut lengthwise into 3 or 4 slices 1 cm wide. Cut these slices into long sticks, also 1 cm wide. Cut the sticks into 3 parts.
2. Season the eggplant sticks with black pepper salt to taste.
3. Spread olive oil and freshly grated cheese. Mix with fingertips until all toothpicks are wrapped in spices.
4. Take them directly to your air fryer basket for 15 minutes at 320^0C.

Nutrition Information

- Calories: 103
- Carbohydrates: 20.98g
- Fat: 0.35g
- Protein: 6.09g
- Sugar: 4.46g
- Cholesterol: 20.98mg

Chapter 8

Air Fryer Dessert Recipes

Australian Chocolate Pie

Servings: 2-3
Preparation time: 5 minutes
Cook time: 5 minutes

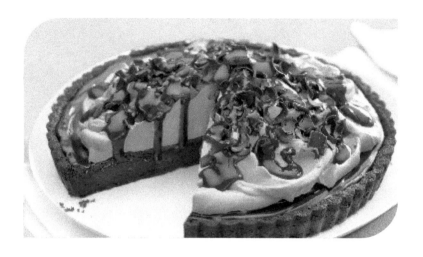

Ingredients

- 1 cup of sugar
- 6 gems
- 1 pound of dark chocolate
- 1 cup of ground almonds
- 2 tbsp of breadcrumbs
- 6 egg whites
- Chocolate glaze
- 1 can of sour cream
  - 1 pound of semi dark chocolate tablets

Steps to Cook

1. Beat the sugar with the egg yolks, add the melted chocolate in a water bath and simply heat.
2. Without stopping to beat, add the almonds and breadcrumbs. Finally, mix the egg whites without hitting them. Pour into a removable pan, greased and lined with foil, also greased, and put in the air fryer for 25 minutes at 400°F. After unmolding and cooling, cover with chocolate icing.

Chocolate glaze:

3. Heat the cream in a double boiler, add the grated chocolate. Stir until fully connected. Let cool a little and cover the cake.

Nutrition Information

- Calories: 241
- Carbohydrates: 26g
- Fat: 13g
- Protein: 3g
- Sugar: 14g
- Cholesterol: 300mg

Australian Brownie

Servings: 2-4
Preparation time: 2 minutes
Cook time: 7 minutes

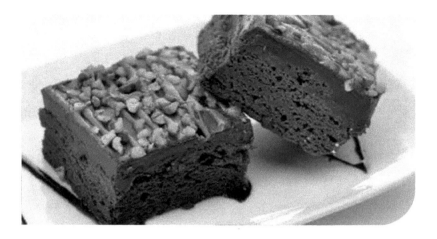

Ingredients

- 1 cup of sugar
- ½ cup all-purpose flour
- 2 eggs
- 1 spoon of vanilla
- ¼ unsalted melted butter
- ½ Cup of powdered chocolate without sugar
- ½ bar of milk chocolate
- 1 cup macadamias, chopped into not too small pieces

Steps to Cook

1. Mix the ingredients in this order until you have a homogeneous mass.
2. Grease a rectangular refractory (that fits in your air fryer).
3. Pour the dough and put it in the air fryer for about 5 to 7 minutes at 350°F.
4. But when testing to stick a toothpick, it should come back clean.
5. Cut into rectangular pieces while still hot.
6. Serve with vanilla ice cream.

Nutrition Information

- Calories: 323
- Carbohydrates: 26.5g
- Fat: 12.8g
- Protein: 3.3g
- Sugar: 17.7g
- Cholesterol: 53mg

Angu Cake

Servings: 4
Preparation time: 30 minutes
Cook time: 15 minutes

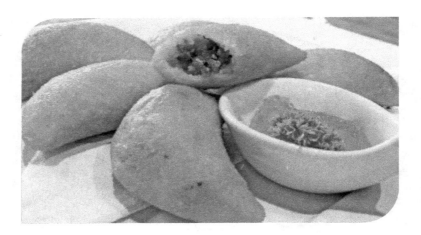

Ingredients

- 4 ¼ cups of water
- 2 tbsp of oil
- 1 tsp salt
- 1 pinch of baking soda
- ½ lb cornmeal
- 1 egg
- ½ cup starch
- ½ lb seasoned and braised ground beef for the filling

Steps to Cook

1. In a frying pan put the water, salt and oil, turn on high heat until it starts to boil, as soon as it starts to boil put the pinch of bicarbonate and pour the cornmeal right away.
2. With a firm spoon, preferably a spoon, stir quickly for about 5 minutes, until it becomes a dough.
3. Place the dough on a bench, open it slightly to cool.
4. Even with the dough from hot to lukewarm, add the egg and the starch and knead well, until obtaining homogeneous and smooth dough.
5. Cover the dough with a plastic or damp cloth so it doesn't dry while modeling the angu cakes.
6. Grab pieces of dough and open them to a thickness of 0.5 cm, cut them with a cutter or pot lid, place the filling in the center and close by joining the two sides of the edges, then press with your fingers to close.
7. You can also model in the hand.
8. Shape all the cakes until the dough and filling are finished, then put them in the Air Fryer basket as many as fit, as shown below.
9. Program the Air Fryer for 15 minutes at 400°F.

10. They will still be clear, but dry on the outside and soft on the inside.

Nutrition Information

- Calories: 60
- Carbohydrates: 8g
- Fat: 1g
- Protein: 2g
- Sugar: 0g
- Cholesterol: 300mg

Cake With Homemade Dough

Servings: 4
Preparation time: 30 minutes
Cook time: 10-12 minutes

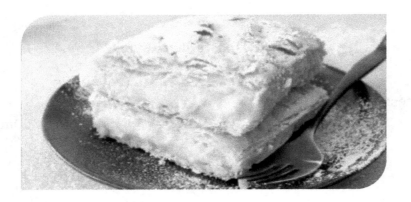

Ingredients

Pasta:
- 1 can of cream
- 2 and 1/3 cups of wheat flour
- 1 teaspoon salt

Steps to Cook

For fillings:
1. Do it to your liking, if it's made of cheese, use firmer cheeses so the dough doesn't explode.

For the dough:
2. In a bowl, mix the cream, flour and salt and knead well to form smooth dough.
1. Use the can with whey and everything and, if you want, you can put it in the Kneading or Dough cycle to beat the bread machine.
2. Once the dough is smooth and smooth, place it in a plastic bag or wrap and let it sit in the refrigerator for 30 minutes. Take the dough out of the refrigerator, take just a piece and spread it out on a smooth surface, about 3ml thick, then cut it to the shape you want, fill it and close it with the tips of a fork on either side of the edges.
3. Place the Air Fryer in a neat monster shape to fit more, and set the Air Fryer for 10-12 minutes at 400°F.

Nutrition Information

- Calories: 323
- Carbohydrates: 26.5g
- Fat: 12.8g
- Protein: 3.3g
- Sugar: 17.7g
- Cholesterol: 53mg

Italian Style Coffee Cake

Servings: 2-4
Preparation time: 10 minutes
Cook time: 20 minutes

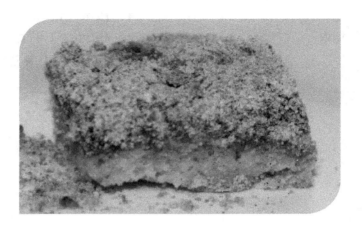

Ingredients

- 6 separate eggs
- 1 cup of sugar
- 2 tbsp of lemon juice
- 1 tbsp grated lemon zest
- 1 tbsp of instant coffee
- 2 tbsp hot water
- ½ cup of ice flour
- 2 tbsp baking powder
- ¼ tbsp of salt

Steps to Cook

1. Beat the egg yolks with the sugar, the juice and the lemon zest. Dissolve the coffee in the hot water.
2. Add to the gems. Sift together the flour, baking powder and salt.
3. Add the egg mixture. Beat the egg whites.
4. Gently add to the dough without mixing too much.
5. Pour the dough into a 22 cm round pan greased and sprinkled with flour.
6. Bake in a preheated oven at 350°F for 20 minutes.
7. Remove from oven and let cool.
8. Cool for 10 minutes before unmolding.
9. Let cool completely.
10. Cover and fill with the coffee cream filling.

Nutrition Information

- Calories: 189
- Carbohydrates: 30g
- Fat: 5.96g
- Protein: 3.51g
- Sugar: 16.62g
- Cholesterol: 55mg

Bean Stew Cookie

Servings: 2-4
Preparation time: 10 minutes
Cook time: 10-15 minutes

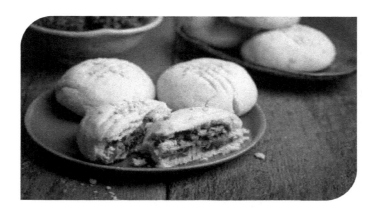

Ingredients

- 3 cups cooked and seasoned black beans or leftover beans with little broth.
- 6 tbsp cassava flour
- 2 tbsp of sour flour

Filling:
- 1 bunch of braised cabbage with cubes of bacon

To bread:
- 1 egg
- 2 cups panko flour, or toasted breadcrumbs.

Steps to Cook

1. For the dough, beat the beans in a blender until it turns into a paste, or use a mixer.
2. Pour the bean paste into a pan and add the yucca flour, stirring well until it turns into a smooth, well-cooked paste.
3. Once warm, add the starch and mix well, set aside and allow cooling completely.
4. To model, take pieces of dough, make a ball, open a dimple in the middle, put the chosen filling and close.
5. After forming the bread, passing the slightly beaten egg and the chosen flour.
6. Place half of the cookies in the Air Fryer basket and adjust for 10-15 minutes at 400°F.

Nutrition Information

- Calories: 65.9
- Carbohydrates: 10.1g
- Fat: 2.4g
- Protein: 1.7g
- Sugar: 4.1g
- Cholesterol: 0.1mg

Chicken Meat Patty

Servings: 2-4
Preparation time: 5 minutes
Cook time: 20-25 minutes

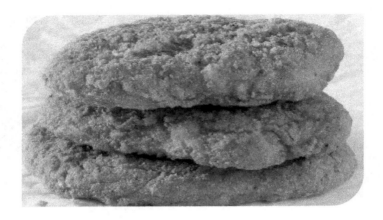

Ingredients

- 1 ½ cup flour
- 1/3 cup butter
- 1 egg
- 3 tbsp parmesan
- ½ tbsp of salt
- ½ tbsp baking powder
- 1 drizzle of olive oil

Filling:

- ½ lb cooked, minced, chicken
- 2 tbsp tomato sauce
- ½ cup cream cheese
- 1/3 can of peas or corn
- 6 chopped olives
- Green aroma to taste

Steps to Cook

1. In a bowl place the flour, butter or margarine, egg white, parmesan, salt and yeast, mix everything until you get smooth and homogeneous dough.
2. Open the dough with a rolling pin or directly into the container to be used, leaving a maximum thickness of 1 cm, then place the already mixed filling and cover with a layer of dough, press firmly on the sides to close the cake and enjoy the nieces of pasta to cut drawings or strips in your cake. Mix the yolk with a drizzle of olive oil and spread on the cake.
3. Place in the Air Fryer basket and program for 20 to 25 minutes at 400°F, until they are very golden.
4. Wait for it to heat up a bit before cutting so as not to break the entire dough and carefully remove it from the Air Fryer so as not to burn.

Nutrition Information

- Calories: 191
- Carbohydrates: 30g
- Fat: 2g
- Protein: 9g
- Sugar: 1g
- Cholesterol: 300mg

Rolled Pizza

Servings: 4
Preparation time: 30 minutes
Cook time: 7 minutes

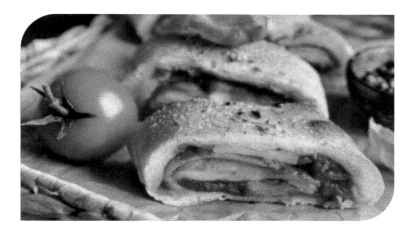

Ingredients

Mass:
- 1 cup warm milk
- 1/3 cup warm water
- ¼ cup olive oil
- 2 tbsp of salt
- 2 tbsp of sugar
- 2 ½ tbsp of yeast
- 4 cups of flour

Filling:
- ½ lb of mozzarella cheese
- 3 ½ oz. of ham
- 1 ½ oz. of sliced olives
- 1/3 cup tomato sauce
- Oregano to taste

Steps to Cook

1. To prepare the dough is very simple, simply mix all the ingredients in a bowl and knead well until you get homogeneous and smooth dough.
2. Be careful not to add flour and make the dough hard, dry, or heavy.
3. If you have a bread machine, just put everything inside the machine shape and set the kneading or dough cycle for at least 30 minutes, then remove and use the dough.
4. Spread the dough out on a smooth rectangular surface, leaving it about 0.5 cm to 1 cm thick.
5. Then add the cheese, the cold cuts, the sauce, the olives and the oregano and roll the dough wide, as shown in the photos below.
6. The filling can be chopped or sliced.
7. Cut the filled dough roll into slices 1.5 cm thick, then place these rolled slices in the Air Fryer basket and adjust for 7 minutes at 400°F.
8. Do this with all the pizzas rolled up until you're done.

Nutrition Information

- Calories: 220
- Carbohydrates: 24g
- Fat: 10g
- Protein: 7g
- Sugar: 3g
- Cholesterol: 10mg

Hot Dog

Servings: 2
Preparation time: 5 minutes
Cook time: 10 minutes

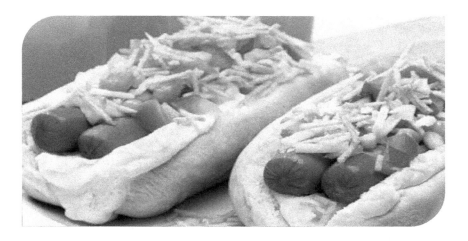

Ingredients

- 2 slices of bread
- 4 sausages
- 4 tbsp of tomato sauce
- 2 medium potatoes
- 1 tbsp butter
- A bit of milk
- Salt
- 4 tbsp grated Parmesan cheese
- Straw potato to serve separately

Steps to Cook

1. Cut the bread into cubes, and then place it in the bottom of the jars or cups.
2. Cut the sausages into slices and mix them with the tomato sauce or the prepared tomato sauce, then divide over the minced bread.
3. Make a firm mash with the boiled mashed potatoes, butter or margarine, salt, and a little milk, and then cover by layering the jars.
4. Place the Parmesan cheese on top. Now place as many jars or cups as you can in the Air Fryer's basket and adjust for 10 minutes at 400°F, until they are golden brown.
10. Serve hot with potatoes at will and be careful not to burn yourself.

Nutrition Information

- Calories: 290
- Carbohydrates: 13g
- Fat: 23g
- Protein: 9g
- Sugar: 4g
- Cholesterol: 300mg

Stuffed Cauliflower

Servings: 2
Preparation time: 15 minutes
Cook time: 10 minutes

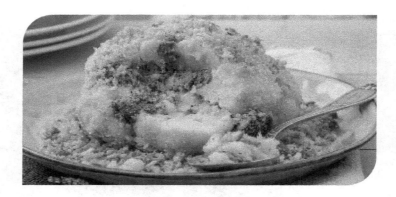

Ingredients

- 1 small or medium cauliflower
- 3 ½ oz. of ham
- 3 ½ oz. of mozzarella
- 1 white sauce recipe
- Parmesan cheese grated to taste

White sauce:

- ½ tbsp of grated onion
- ½ tbsp minced garlic
- 1 tbsp butter
- 1 tbsp of wheat flour
- 2 pinches of salt
- 1 pinch of nutmeg
- 1 ½ cups milk

Steps to Cook

1. Cut the cauliflower into bouquets, wash well, then place in a pan and cover with water, add ½ teaspoon of salt and a few drops of vinegar.
2. Cook over high heat until tender and cooked through.
3. Do not cover the pan during cooking as the water may overflow.
4. Meanwhile, prepare the white sauce.
5. In a frying pan put the butter or margarine, onion and garlic, as soon as the margarine melts add the flour immediately and stir well until it turns into clay.
6. Then add the milk little by little without stopping, until it turns into a cream with the texture of the sauce.
7. Add the nutmeg and salt, and then the sauce is ready.
8. If you don't have much practice, you can beat all the sauce ingredients in a blender and then bring to medium heat, stirring constantly until the point is in the sauce.
9. Separate a container that can enter the Air Fryer.
10. Put a little sauce in the bottom of the pan, then the cauliflower already drained, between the cauliflower bouquets, place and sink pieces of cheese and ham,

then cover with the rest of the sauce and the Parmesan cheese al taste.

11. Adjust the Air Fryer for 10 minutes at 400°F, until it is golden brown, depending on your taste, you can leave more time.

Nutrition Information

- Calories: 104.1
- Carbohydrates: 7.6g
- Fat: 8g
- Protein: 2.1g
- Sugar: 1.3g
- Cholesterol: 21.1mg

Sequilho

Servings: 50
Preparation time: 5 minutes
Cook time: 10-12 minutes

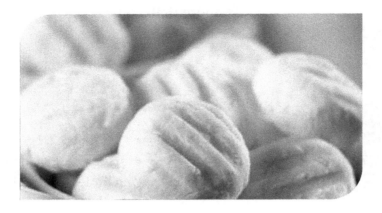

Ingredients

- 1 package of onion soup powder
- 2 cups of wheat flour
- ½ cup margarine or butter
- 1 egg
- 1 tbsp grated Parmesan cheese
- 2 tbsp of water
- 1 tbsp of baking powder

Steps to Cook

1. In a bowl, put all the ingredients together and mix well, until it reaches the similar point of rotten, i.e., brittle, dough that is firm but not elastic and breaks slightly when squeezed.
2. Roll the dough and squeeze with a fork to flatten and mark.
3. Place half of the cookies in the Air Fryer basket and place them for 10 to 12 minutes at 400°F, they should be golden.
4. Remove from Air Fryer and allow to cool, place the other half of the cookies and repeat the process.
5. Once ready, before storage, after cold, they can be stored for up to 15 days in a closed container.

Nutrition Information

- Calories: 53
- Carbohydrates: 7.3g
- Fat: 2.04g
- Protein: 1.24g
- Sugar: 0.07g
- Cholesterol: 0mg

Fried Polenta

Servings: 2-4
Preparation time: 5 minutes
Cook time: 18 minutes

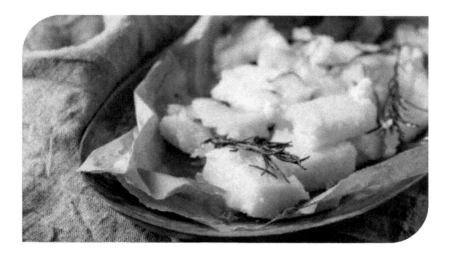

Ingredients

- 3 cups of tea
- 1 sachet or tablet of chicken or vegetable broth
- 1 tbsp butter
- 1 tsp of shallow salt
- 1 cup plain or precooked cornmeal

Steps to Cook

1. Put the water, the broth, the butter or the margarine and the salt in a frying pan and bring to the fire, when it begins to boil, sprinkle the cornmeal over the water, stirring constantly, until the cornmeal is finished. Keep stirring well with a spoon. Stir very quickly and without stopping.
2. Lower the heat to avoid splashing and stir until it begins to free from the bottom of the pan, this takes up to 10 minutes, but if you use a good cornmeal or the precooked cornmeal is super fast, only about 3-5 minutes.
3. When it gets to the point, to release from the bottom of the pan, pour it into a greased baking dish with butter or margarine, spread it out well and let it heat or cool, then it will harden so you can cut it with a knife about 2 cm wide.
4. Place the polenta next to each other in the Air Fryer for 18 minutes at 400°F and they are ready.

Nutrition Information

- Calories: 77
- Carbohydrates: 16.24g
- Fat: 0.35g
- Protein: 1.77g
- Sugar: 0.13g
- Cholesterol: 0mg

Churros Filled With Caramel

Servings: 20
Preparation time: 10 minutes
Cook time: 21 minutes

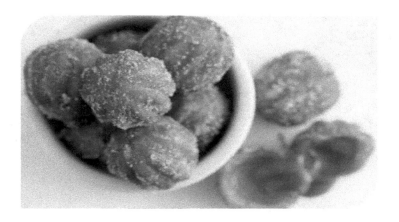

Ingredients

Caramel:
- 1 cup of dulce de leche
- ½ cup whole milk

Churros:
- 1 cup of wheat flour
- 1 cup cornmeal
- ½ tsp of baking soda
- ½ tsp baking powder
- 2 cups of cold water
- 1 pinch of salt
- 2 tbsp of canola oil
- 2 tbsp of sugar

To sprinkle:
- ½ cup of tea
- 1 tsp ground cinnamon

Steps to Cook

1. For the syrup, heat the dulce de leche and add the milk. Mix well and let stand.
2. For churros, preheat the Air fryer to 400°F for 3 minutes. Mix dry ingredients (except salt and sugar) and set aside. Put water, salt, oil, and sugar in a saucepan and bring to a boil.
3. Incorporate the dry ingredients into the pan, mixing vigorously. Cook for 3 minutes over medium heat.
4. Place the dough in a pastry bag with a hole of about 1.5 cm. Make the churros about 8 cm long.
5. Place the churros in the Air fryer for 10 minutes, rotating them when you complete 5 minutes.
6. Wrap the churros in the sugar and cinnamon mixture.

Nutrition Information

- Calories: 291.5
- Carbohydrates: 66.7g
- Fat: 0.3g
- Protein: 7.9g
- Sugar: 2.3g
- Cholesterol: 45mg

Bisnaguinha Gluten Free Bread

Servings: 2-4
Preparation time: 5 minutes
Cook time: 10 minutes

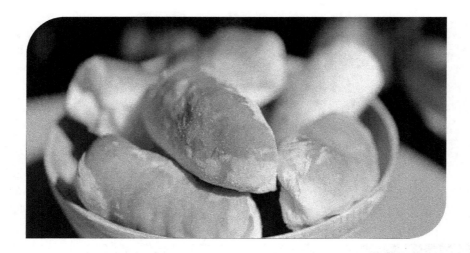

Ingredients

- 1/3 lb of rice flour
- 2 oz. of potato starch
- 1 ½ oz sweet powder
- 1 tbsp xanthan gum
- 1 tsp baking powder
- 1 ½ oz. of honey
- 1 pinch of salt
- ½ cup of warm milk
- 2 oz. plain yogurt
- 1 ¼ oz. margarine, softened

Steps to Cook

1. In a bowl, mix together the flour, salt, and yeast.
2. Mix the remaining ingredients until they form smooth and homogeneous dough, which does not adhere to your hands. If the dough is too dry, add more yogurts to the point. Divide the dough into 9 balls.
3. Cover with a cloth and let it grow for at least 30 minutes. If you want it to be golden, brush the egg on top before baking. Remove the flat basket from the fryer and preheat the fryer for 5 minutes at 350°F. Line the fryer bowl with parchment paper and carefully place the balls inside the bowl, leaving a possible space between them.
4. Set 20 minutes to 350°F. Stick with a toothpick to see if it's ready, if it's still damp inside, allow more time.

Nutrition Information

- Calories: 126
- Carbohydrates: 23g
- Fat: 3.2g
- Protein: 2.4g
- Sugar: 0g
- Cholesterol: 0mg

Salty French Toast

Servings: 2-4
Preparation time: 5 minutes
Cook time: 6-8 minutes

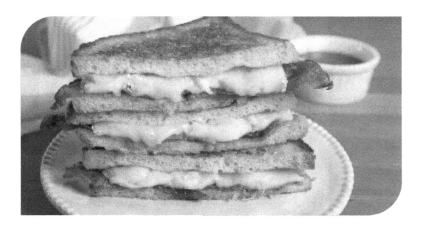

Ingredients

- 3 French breads
- 1 cup milk
- 1/3 cup creamy cottage cheese
- 1 pinch of salt
- 1 pinch of oregano and/or other herbs of your choice
- 1 drizzle of olive oil
- 2 eggs
- ½ lb grated parmesan, can be thin or thick

Steps to Cook

1. In a bowl mix the milk, the curd, the salt, the herbs and the olive oil, if the milk is warm it is easier to mix.
2. In another bowl place the two eggs and beat lightly, and in another bowl place the grated cheese, which can also be added with herbs to your liking.
3. Cut the bread into slices about 2 to 3 centimeters thick.
4. Dip each slice of bread into the milk mixture, then the beaten eggs and finally the grated Parmesan cheese.
5. Place one slice side by side in the Air Fryer's basket as in the images below.
6. Program from 6 to 8 minutes at 400°F.

Nutrition Information

- Calories: 218
- Carbohydrates: 22.9g
- Fat: 5.8g
- Protein: 19.7g
- Sugar: 5.5g
- Cholesterol: 186mg

Sausage Braid

Servings: 2-4
Preparation time: 5 minutes
Cook time: 25 minutes

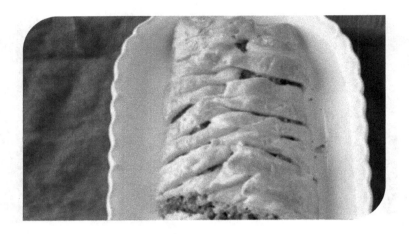

Ingredients

Dough:
- cup of warm milk
- ¼ cup olive oil or olive oil
- 2 tsp of salt
- 2 tbsp of sugar
- 2 ½ tsp of yeast
- 4 cups of wheat flour

Filling:
- 8 to 10 sausages or thin smoked sausages

Steps to Cook

1. For the dough just mix all the ingredients in a bowl and knead well until you get a smooth and homogeneous dough. Be careful not to add too much flour and make the dough hard or heavy.
2. After the dough is ready, separate the pieces and open them to a thickness of about 0.5 cm, put the sausage in the middle, roll up and cut the excess dough from the sides.
3. cut the sausage wrapped in the dough into slices of about 1 cm, but without reaching the end of the dough, now just pull it to the side by turning it slightly and repeat the process with all the slices, from side to side and each other to the end.
4. After shaping, place it in the Air Fryer basket and program it for 8 minutes at 350°F.

Nutrition Information

- Calories: 285
- Carbohydrates: 3.5g
- Fat: 22.7g
- Protein: 15.9g
- Sugar: 0.7g
- Cholesterol: 47m

Super Burger

Servings: 20
Preparation time: 5 minutes
Cook time: 1h 30 minutes

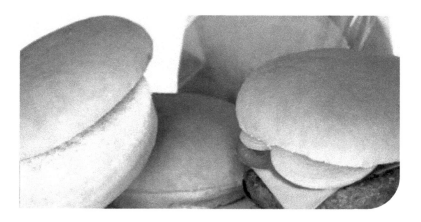

Ingredients

Mass:
- 1 cup warm milk
- 1/3 cup warm water
- ¼ cup olive oil
- 2 tbsp of salt
- 2 tbsp of sugar
- 2 ½ tbsp of yeast
- 4 cups of flour

Filling:
- 8 fried burgers
- 250 g of cheddar cheese or plate
- Ceiling
- 1 egg yolk to brush
- 1 tablespoon of sesame

Steps to Cook

1. Mix all the ingredients of the dough in a bowl and knead well until smooth and homogeneous.
2. Be careful not to add flour and make the dough hard, dry, or heavy.
3. Prepared dough and fried and cold burgers, let's model the burgers.
4. Divide the dough into 8 equal parts, make a ball with each part of the dough, then open each dough by hand or with a rolling pin, place two slices of cheese in the center and on top of the hamburger.
5. Close by pulling the edges to the center and then lower.
6. Brush with yolk and sprinkle with sesame to decorate.
7. Place 2 hamburgers in the Air Fryer basket and program for 12 minutes at 350°F. Repeat the process with the others and enjoy.

Nutrition Information

- Calories: 564
- Carbohydrates: 27g
- Fat: 38g
- Protein: 26 g
- Sugar: 14g
- Cholesterol: 89mg

Soufflé

Servings: 2-4
Preparation time: 30 minutes
Cook time: 15 minutes

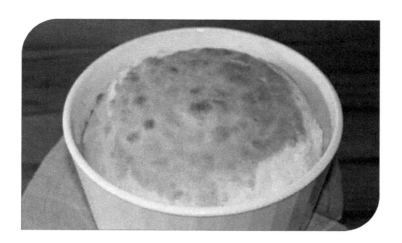

Ingredients

- 2 tbsp of wheat flour
- 1 cup milk
- 1 tbsp butter
- 1 pinch of salt
- 1 tbsp of grated cheese
- 3 eggs
- Green smell to taste
- 1 cup of the chosen filling

Steps to Cook

1. In a frying pan put the flour, butter or margarine, milk and salt, mix well and light the fire, keep stirring until a cream is formed, then add the filling of your choice, the green smell and the egg yolks and stir well until well mixed.
2. Meanwhile, beat the egg whites and then add to the mixture you made in the pan, gradually and stirring gently so as not to lose the sweetness of the whites.
3. Separate 4 molds or porcelain or ceramic molds and grease with olive oil.
4. Place 2 jars in the Air Fryer at the same time, for 15 minutes at 400°F.

Nutrition Information

- Calories: 270
- Carbohydrates: 7.4g
- Fat: 11g
- Protein: 16g
- Sugar: 2.9g
- Cholesterol: 196mg

Pine Nut Balls

Servings: 30
Preparation time: 15 mins
Cook time: 10 minutes

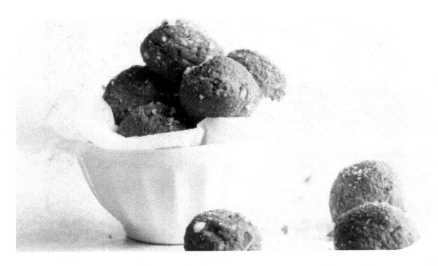

Ingredients

- 2 cups of pine nuts cooked and peeled
- 1 cup cooked rice
- 1 large egg
- 1 tbsp of wheat flour
- 1 tbsp of olive oil
- 1 tbsp of onion
- 1 tbsp of garlic
- 2 tbsp of grated cheese
- Salt
- Black pepper
- Parsley and chives to
- ½ cup of filling to your liking

Steps to Cook

1. Separate the filling of your choice.
2. In the food processor, place the pinion and whisk until chopped, then add all other ingredients including the chosen filling and whisk until you see it ignite.
3. Roll this dough into balls, if it sticks stick a little oil on your hands.
4. Place the balls in the Air Fryer basket and adjust for 10 minutes at 400°F, if you want more golden brownies, leave a few more minutes..

Nutrition Information

- Calories: 40.4
- Carbohydrates: 0.8g
- Fat: 4.1g
- Protein: 0.8g
- Sugar: 0.2g
- Cholesterol: 0mg

Blender cake

Servings: 4-6
Preparation time: 5 minutes
Cook time: 25 minutes

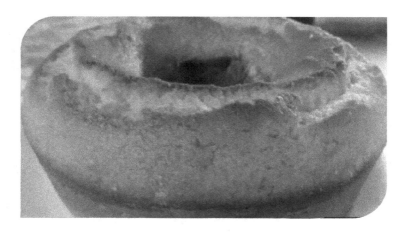

Ingredients

- 1 cup milk
- 1 egg
- 1 tbsp of olive oil or olive oil
- 1 tbsp butter
- 1 tbsp of grated cheese
- 1 pinch of salt
- 1 cup all-purpose flour
- 1 tsp of yeast

Filling:

- 1 cup of filling of your choice.

Steps to Cook

1. Put all the ingredients of the dough in the blender in the previous order, beat for 1 minute, just to mix practically. Pour half of the dough into the container you are going to use, already greased with olive oil, oil, butter or margarine.
2. Place the filling of your choice, leaving a border of at least 1 cm on the sides so that the dough closes when baking.
3. Then pour the rest of the dough on top.
4. Program the Air Fryer for 25 minutes at 400°F.
5. Stick with a toothpick to see if it's already baked after about 20 minutes. If the toothpick comes out clean, it's ready.
6. Expect to heat, unmold, and serve.

Nutrition Information

- Calories: 650
- Carbohydrates: 74g
- Fat: 37g
- Protein: 8g
- Sugar: 61g
- Cholesterol: 195mg

Zucchini Soufflé With Cheese And Ham

Servings: 2-4
Preparation time: 10 mins
Cook time: 45 minutes

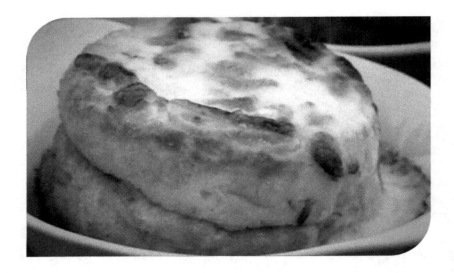

Ingredients

- 4 beaten eggs
- 1 small zucchini in strips
- ½ can of cream
- 1 tbsp cornstarch
- 1 tbsp baking powder
- 3 slices of ham in strips
- 3 slices of mozzarella in strips
- Oregano and salt to taste

Steps to Cook

1. Beat the eggs, add the other ingredients.
2. Grease the pan and pour the mixture.
3. Bake in 30 minutes with a temperature of 160° in the first 15 minutes and then increase to 350°F.
4. Serve immediately.

Nutrition Information

- Calories: 278.8
- Carbohydrates: 12.2g
- Fat: 17.5g
- Protein: 17.8g
- Sugar: 0.6g
- Cholesterol: 65.2mg

Hot Canape

Servings: 6
Preparation time: 5 minutes
Cook time: 5 minutes

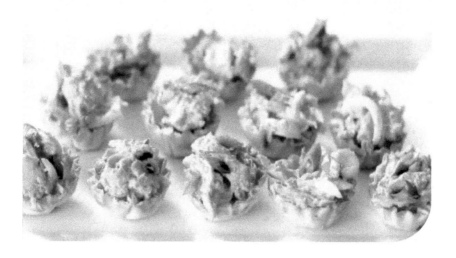

Ingredients

- Loaf of bread or small toast
- Cottage cheese or cream cheese
- Other coatings to your liking

Steps to Cook

1. Prepare the toast with a layer of cottage cheese or cream cheese and place it in the fryer basket without oil.
2. If you use a loaf of bread, cut it into small pieces to facilitate the accommodation in the basket and to vary the ingredients.
3. Add the topping of your choice, such as chicken, cheese, olives, deli meats, and general sausages.
4. Set from 3 to 5 minutes at 400°F, the time varies according to the bread used, the intention is to make it golden

Nutrition Information

- Calories: 166.6
- Carbohydrates: 19.5g
- Fat: 2.4g
- Protein: 3.9g
- Sugar: 0.7g
- Cholesterol: 20.7mg

Cheese Fondue

Servings: 2-4
Preparation time: 5 minutes
Cook time: 8 minutes

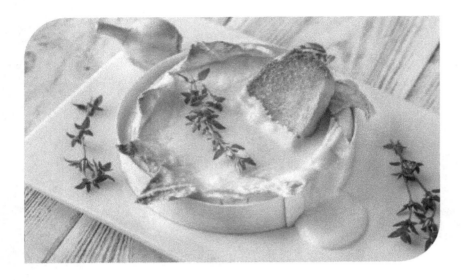

Ingredients

- ½ lb of grated mozzarella
- ½ lb of grated provolone
- 4 tbsp grated parmesan
- 1 can of cream

Steps to Cook

1. In a refractory container, mix all the cheeses with the cream, arrange them well, and then place them in the Air Fryer basket.
2. Program the Air Fryer for 25 minutes at 400°F or 180°C if you want it well gratinated.

Nutrition Information

- Calories: 144
- Carbohydrates: 0.8g
- Fat: 9.2g
- Protein: 8.5g
- Sugar: 0.3g
- Cholesterol: 31mg

Lasagna

Servings: 4
Preparation time: 5 minutes
Cook time: 25 minutes

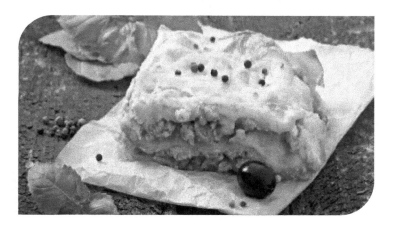

Ingredients

- 1 package of lasagna pasta
- 1 can of tomato sauce
- ½ lb of ham
- ½ lb of mozzarella
- grated fresh parmesan cheese

Steps to Cook

1. In a bowl of water, place the lasagna dough one by one and leave it for 5 minutes. Now in the closed form of the air fryer, not the one with holes is another one that goes inside the holes.
2. Let's start the assembly in the closed basket. Make a light layer of sauce, then make a layer with the dough, if necessary break a little dough. Then make a layer of sauce, a layer of mozzarella and a layer of ham
3. Repeat the process until you finish with a layer of pasta and the sauce on top. Finish with grated Parmesan.
4. Heat the air fryer for 3 minutes at 320°F. Then place the closed pan inside the basket with holes in the fryer. Set the timer for 17 minutes at 320°F.

Nutrition Information

- Calories: 440
- Carbohydrates: 10.5g
- Fat: 21.2g
- Protein: 25.1g
- Sugar: 0g
- Cholesterol: 103mg

Amazing Condensed Milk Pudding

Servings: 2
Preparation time: 20 minutes
Cook time: 1h30 minutes

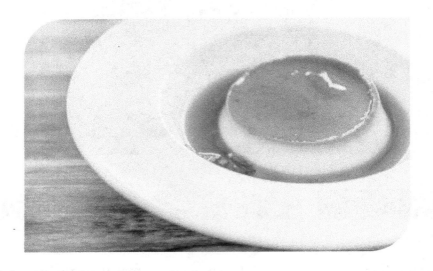

Ingredients

- 6 eggs
- 5 oz. of sugar
- 1 tsp of vanilla
- 1 lb condensed milk
- 1 ¼ cup milk

Steps to Cook

1. Let's prepare the caramel. The challenge is to do absolutely everything in the fryer, so you can make the caramel on the air fryer if you want.
2. You can choose to make caramel on the stove as well.
3. Put the sugar in the pan and add 8 tablespoons of water of sugar equals about 7 tablespoons of sugar, so use a tablespoon of water more than sugar, follow this ratio if you want more syrup.
4. Mix well and place in air fryer for 18 to 23 min at 390°F.
5. Just note the candy color once in a while, don't make it too dark.
6. You do not need to stir the sugar, it is ready on its own.
7. In a bowl, add 2 whole eggs and 4 yolks. Mix with a fork.
8. Add the condensed milk, milk and vanilla.

9. Mix well.
10. With the syrup ready, it's time to grease the pan with it.
11. The shape will come out very hot, so be careful.
1. Using a silicone brush, brush the entire side and center until it forms a good layer of caramel.
2. This is very important to unmold the milk pudding.
3. Using a sieve, fill the pan with the reserved dough. By sifting, we will remove any film from the eggs and leave the pudding soft.
4. Pack the pudding shape with aluminum foil, close the sides tightly.
5. Place to roast in the electric fryer from 1h to 1: 30h at 230°F.
6. Every 30 minutes, open the fryer to get some heat out. Just pull out the drawer, wait 20 seconds and put it back in.

Nutrition Information

- Calories: 255.8
- Carbohydrates: 37.5g
- Fat: 8g
- Protein: 7.6g
- Sugar: 26.8g
- Cholesterol: 103.8mg

American Toast With Fried Egg In The Middle

Servings: 2-4
Preparation time: 2 minutes
Cook time: 7 minutes

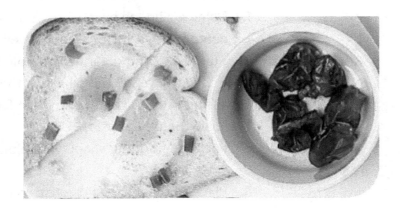

Ingredients

- 1 whole Egg
- 1 slice of bread
- Salt and pepper to taste
- Chicken to taste

Steps to Cook

1. Make a circular, square, heart-shaped cut or any other shape you want in the center of the bread and remove the leftovers.
2. Separate the egg into a small container for easy handling.
3. Preheat the fryer for 3 minutes at 320°F.
4. Whimsical in the decoration of the dish, dried cherry tomatoes are a very tasty accompaniment to this toast, they also serve a juice of fresh and colorful fruits. This is an addictive, tasty and fun recipe for adults and children.

Nutrition Information

- Calories: 542.9
- Carbohydrates: 48.2g
- Fat: 30.6g
- Protein: 20.4g
- Sugar: 0.8g
- Cholesterol: 451mg

Fried Aubergine Breading A Milanesa

Servings: 2
Preparation time: 10 minutes
Cook time: 3 minutes

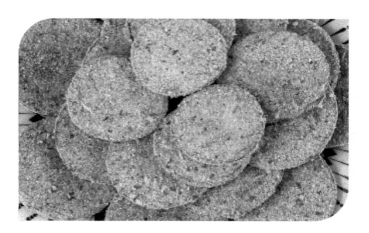

Ingredients

- 1 large eggplant
- 2 oz. breadcrumbs
- 1 spoon of dehydrated parsley soup
- 1 parmesan soup spoon
- 1 egg
- salt and pepper to taste

Steps to Cook

1. Cut the eggplant into thin slices. Ours produced 21 slices. Beat the egg well until smooth between the white and the yolk. Mix the Parmesan cheese, dried parsley, salt and pepper with breadcrumbs. Mix the Parmesan cheese, dried parsley, salt and pepper with breadcrumbs. It is also possible to make with cornmeal, but the color will not be very appetizing.
2. Preheat the fryer for 3 minutes at 350°F. Arrange the slices in the basket in layers, drizzle olive oil and continue to arrange with a new layer of aubergines and drizzle again. Fill only with two layers of eggplant.

Nutrition Information

- Calories: 60
- Carbohydrates: 8g
- Fat: 1g
- Protein: 2g
- Sugar: 0g
- Cholesterol: 300mg

Homemade French Toast

Servings: 2-4
Preparation time: 15 minutes
Cook time: 8 minutes

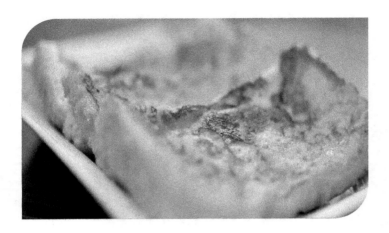

Ingredients

- stale French bread slices or toast
- 1 egg
- 1 cup of milk
- 1 can of condensed milk
- Sugar
- Cinnamon

Steps to Cook

1. Mix egg, milk and condensed milk. Roll the slices of bread into this mixture. Then roll them in mixed sugar and cinnamon. Place the bread in the Air Fryer's basket and turn it on, leaving it for approximately 8 minutes at 390°F.
2. There, your French toast will be wonderful!
3. If desired, when you remove it from the Air Fryer, you can sprinkle icing sugar.

Nutrition Information

- Calories: 200
- Carbohydrates: 31g
- Fat: 6g
- Protein: 10g
- Sugar: 5g
- Cholesterol: 285mg

Coffee Cake

Servings: 1-2
Preparation time: 10 minutes
Cook time: 15 minutes

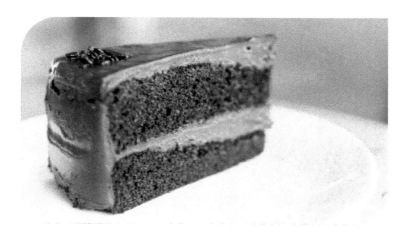

Ingredients

- 4 tbsp of wheat flour
- 4 tbsp of sugar
- 2 tbsp of powdered chocolate
- 2 tbsp baking powder
- 1 unit of egg
- 3 tbsp of milk
- 3 tbsp of soybean oil

Steps to Cook

1. Put the flour, chocolate and sugar in the cup.
2. Mix with a fork. Add the egg and mix again.
3. Put the milk and oil. Mixture.
4. Preheat your fryer for 5 min.
5. Bring to the fryer for 15 minutes at 320°F.

Note: You can add a syrup or topping of your choice to make it taste better!

Nutrition Information

- Calories: 189
- Carbohydrates: 30g
- Fat: 5.96g
- Protein: 3.51g
- Sugar: 16.62g
- Cholesterol: 55mg

Chocolate Molten Lava Cake

Servings: 2-4
Preparation time: 10 minutes
Cook time: 10 minutes

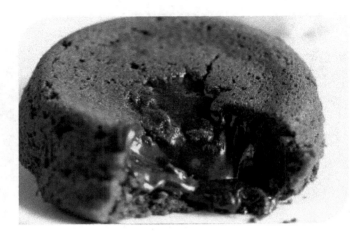

Ingredients

- 6 tbsp unsalted butter cut into pieces
- 4 oz semi-sweet chocolate bar broken into pieces
- 1 large egg
- 1 egg yolk from a large egg
- 3 tbsp of white sugar
- ½ tsp of vanilla extract
- 2 tbsp all-purpose flour
- pinch of salt

Steps to Cook

1. Grease 3 6-ounce molds and set aside.
2. Melt the butter and chocolate in a microwave-safe bowl for about 1 minute until melted, stirring every 30 seconds. Set aside.
3. In a separate large bowl, use an electric mixer and beat the egg, egg yolk, vanilla extract, and sugar until well blended.
4. Then add the flour, chocolate mixture and a pinch of salt and stir until combined. Pour the mixture into the molds, filling each half.
5. Place in the fryer basket and air fry at 370^0 F for 8-10 minutes.
6. Once you are done frying, use a clean, thick kitchen towel to remove the molds from the fryer basket. Let the cake cool in a pan for about 1 minute. Use a butter knife to loosen the cake from the pan and flip it onto a plate. Serve with fresh whipped cream, fresh berries or powdered sugar and enjoy.

Nutrition Information

- Calories: 660
- Carbohydrates: 66g
- Fat: 41g
- Protein: 10g
- Sugar: 47g
- Cholesterol: 304mg

Petit Gateau

Servings: 2-4
Preparation time: 5 minutes
Cook time: 10 minutes

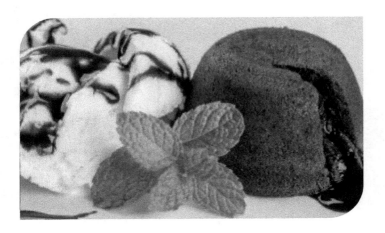

Ingredients

- 6 tbsp unsalted butter
- 5 ¼ oz. of chopped dark chocolate
- 1 large egg
- 1 egg yolk
- 3 spoonfuls of sugar
- ½ tbsp vanilla extract
- 2 tbsp of wheat flour
- 1 pinch of salt

Steps to Cook

1. Grease 3 molds and reserve.
2. Melt butter and chocolate in a microwaveable bowl for about 1 minute until melted, stirring every 30 seconds. Reserve.
3. In a large bowl, use an electric mixer and beat the eggs, yolk, vanilla extract, and sugar until well blended. Then add the flour, chocolate mixture and a pinch of salt and stir until combined. Pour the mixture into the molds, filling each half.
4. Place in the fryer basket and bake at 350°F for 8-10 minutes.
5. Remove molds from fryer basket. Let the cake cool in a pan for about 1 minute. Use a butter knife to drop the cake pan into a plate. Serve with a scoop of ice cream and enjoy.

Nutrition Information

- Calories: 66
- Carbohydrates: 6g
- Fat: 4g
- Protein: 1g
- Sugar: 14g
- Cholesterol: 300mg

Sweet Cookie With Coco

Servings: 4
Preparation time: 30 minutes
Cook time: 7 minutes

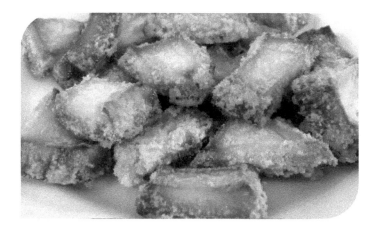

Ingredients

- 1 dry coconut
- ½ cup of refined sugar tea
- 100 ml of water

Steps to Cook

1. Remove the water from the dried coconut. Remove the dried coconut shell. And for that, place it inside the basket of the electric fryer, turn on the fryer and keep it at a temperature of 390^0F for 15 minutes.
2. With the help of a silicone glove or a thermal glove, remove the coconut from the fryer.
3. With the help of a hammer, break the rest of the skin. You will see that the coconut pulp will be very loose.
4. Cut the coconut into small pieces.
5. Dampen these pieces with water and skim the refined sugar, like you're shaking the coconut.
6. Distribute these pieces into the basket of the air fryer. Try not to put one on top of the other. Leave well spread.
7. Keep the fryer at 390°F for a period that can vary from 10 to 15 minutes. During this time, open the air fryer and check the coconut until they begin to brown.
8. Remove the sweet coconuts from the air frying pan and let them cool.

Nutrition Information

- Calories: 137
- Carbohydrates: 19g
- Fat: 6.4g
- Protein: 1.3g
- Sugar: 12g
- Cholesterol: 21mg

Sweet Corn Cake With Guava Pasta

Servings: 2-4
Preparation time: 15 minutes
Cook time: 35 minutes

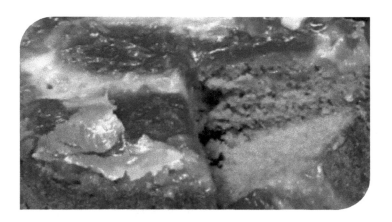

Ingredients

- 1 cup cassava
- 1 cup brown sugar
- 2 tbsp of flour
- 1 tbsp ground cinnamon
- 1 egg
- ¼ cup of oil
- 1 tbsp butter
- ½ tbsp baking powder
- 2 tbsp refined sugar
- ½ cup milk
- ½ cup of cottage cheese
- guava strips to taste

Steps to Cook

1. Separate the yolk from the white.
2. Beat the egg whites; sweeten with refined sugar and reserve.
3. Cover the bottom of the pan with curd and place a layer of guava strips.
4. Beat the remaining ingredients in a blender or mixer.
5. Add the yeast and mix.
6. Add the egg white and mix with a spoon.
7. Pour mixture into a round nonstick or oiled skillet that will fit in the fryer.
8. With the air fryer already preheated to 5 minutes, set it for 35 minutes at a temperature between 572°F and 608°F.
11. After cooling, turn the plate onto a plate and serve.

Nutrition Information

- Calories: 259
- Carbohydrates: 30g
- Fat: 15g
- Protein: 3g
- Sugar: 11g
- Cholesterol: 31mg

Layered Apple Pie

Servings: 2
Preparation time: 15 minutes
Cook time: 20 minutes

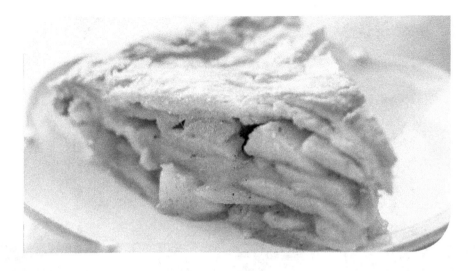

Ingredients

- 3 unpeeled apples, thinly sliced
- 1 cup all-purpose flour
- 1 cup of sugar
- 1 tbsp ground cinnamon
- 1 cup milk
- 1 tbsp unsalted melted butter
- 1 egg
- 1 tbsp vanilla essence

Steps to Cook

1. Mix the flour, sugar and cinnamon. Reserve.
2. Lightly beat the egg with a fork, add the milk, vanilla and melted butter. Reservation.
3. In the container that comes with the Air fryer, make thin layers, alternating apple slices and dry ingredients. Finish with a dry coat. Finally, carefully pour the liquid mixture over everything and take it to the Air fryer for 20 minutes at 250°F.

Nutrition Information

- Calories: 413
- Carbohydrates: 78g
- Fat: 11g
- Protein: 3.7g
- Sugar: 51g
- Cholesterol: 0.1mg

Tortilla Caprese

Servings: 2-4
Preparation time: 1 minute
Cook time: 10 minutes

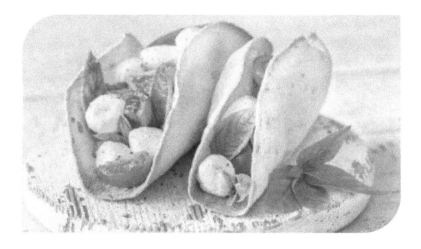

Ingredients

- 6 tomatoes cut in half, seasoned with oil, salt and pepper
- Basil leaves (to taste)
- 1 unit of cubed cheese
- 3 beaten eggs with a pinch of salt

Steps to Cook

1. In the container that comes with the Air fryer, place the cheese and tomatoes. Add the eggs and basil leaves. Take Air fryer for 10 minutes at 180°F.

Nutrition Information

- Calories: 234.7
- Carbohydrates: 26.9g
- Fat: 9.2g
- Protein: 12.7g
- Sugar: 1g
- Cholesterol: 10mg

German Garlic Bread

Servings: 2-3
Preparation time: 10 mins
Cook time: 10 minutes

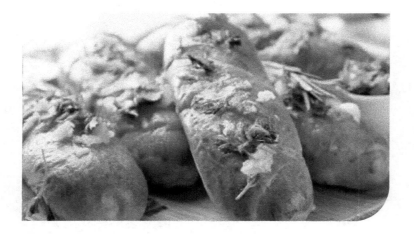

Ingredients

- 3 stale French rolls
- 4 tbsp of crushed garlic
- 1 cup butter
- Grated Parmesan cheese for sprinkling
- 1 tbsp of olive oil

Steps to Cook

1. Preheat an electric fryer to 390°F, until the green light comes on.
2. Mix the butter or margarine with the garlic and set aside.
3. With the help of a brush, spread the oil over the rolls.
4. Cut the rolls into slices, but without separating them completely, and distribute the garlic paste in the cavities, evenly.
5. Close the rolls, sprinkle with the grated Parmesan cheese, and place them in the basket on the electric fryer.
6. Set the fryer for 10 minutes and set the temperature to 350°F. At the end of time, your garlic breads will be ready to serve.

Nutrition Information

- Calories: 53
- Carbohydrates: 7.3g
- Fat: 2.04g
- Protein: 1.24g
- Sugar: 0.07g
- Cholesterol: 0mg

Wholemeal Bread With Egg Curry

Servings: 20
Preparation time: 10 minutes
Cook time: 21 minutes

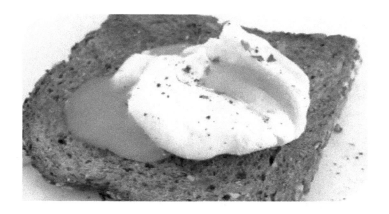

Ingredients

- 2 slices of bread
- 1 unit of raw chicken egg
- ½ tsp full of curry

Steps to Cook

1. Using a cup, punch a hole in the middle of one of the bread slices and remove this crumb, lay it on top of the other slice and microwave, quickly break one egg in the center and lay it for 30 seconds. Season with curry and salt and pierce the yolk, take it to the micro for another 30 seconds. To make it crispy, take it to the air fryer for 3 minutes at 230^0F. Use the crumb as a garnish.

Nutrition Information

- Calories: 266.6
- Carbohydrates: 2.4g
- Fat: 9.4g
- Protein: 9.6g
- Sugar: 0g
- Cholesterol: 102.1mg

Bread Lasagna And White Sauce

Servings: 4-6
Preparation time: 5 minutes
Cook time: 30 minutes

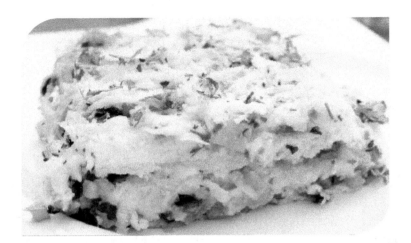

Ingredients

- 1 package loaf of bread
- 1 lb of ham
- 1 lb mozzarella cheese
- 3 ½ oz. parmesan
- 2 cups milk
- 2 tbsp cornstarch dissolved in ½ glass of water
- 1 tbsp of margarine
- 1 onion, finely chopped
- 1 bacon broth or your choice
- 1 can of cream

Steps to Cook

White sauce:
1. Fry the onion in the margarine until golden. Bring the milk and bacon broth to a boil. Add cornstarch and stir until thick. Turn off the heat and add the cream.

Assemblage:
2. In a refractory or greased rectangular pan, place 6 slices of bread. Sprinkle with a ladle of white sauce and spread well over the slices. Add a layer of ham, another layer of cheese, and sprinkle with grated cheese. Change the layers again. Finish with the ham and mozzarella. Throw the remaining white cream over the entire loaf, with plenty.
3. Sprinkle with Parmesan cheese and bring to the air fryer for 30 minutes at 350°F.

Nutrition Information

- Calories: 353.5
- Carbohydrates: 32.1g
- Fat: 16g
- Protein: 19.1g
- Sugar: 4.5g
- Cholesterol: 119.7mg

Portuguese Flatbread Pizza

Servings: 4-6
Preparation time: 5 minutes
Cook time: 25 minutes

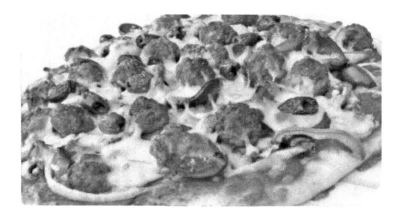

Ingredients

- 1 package of loaf of bread
- 1 box of tomato sauce
- ½ lb of cheese
- ½ lb of ham
- 2 cans of grated tuna or sardine puree
- 1 can of corn with peas
- 1 onion, sliced
- 1 tomato, sliced
- 2 boiled eggs, sliced
- Olive to taste
- Olive oil
- Oregano

Steps to Cook

4. Remove the breadcrumbs and flatten them with a rolling pin
5. Grease a pan with oil and place the loaves.
1. Then pass the tomato sauce without leaving space, but do not over-dry.
2. Place the cheese to spread without holes, the ham in the same way.
3. Grated tuna or sardines, and the corn and pea duet spread well.
4. Spread onion rings, tomato slices, eggs, olives and drizzle on top with a little olive oil.
5. Finally the oregano.
6. Put in the preheated air fryer at 320°F for 25 minutes, let the cheese melt and the bread is crisp on the bottom.

Nutrition Information

- Calories: 130
- Carbohydrates: 26.32g
- Fat: 0.57g
- Protein: 4.3g
- Sugar: 0.61g
- Cholesterol: 0mg

Zucchini Bolognese Lasagna

Servings: 2-4
Preparation time: 5 minutes
Cook time: 15 minutes

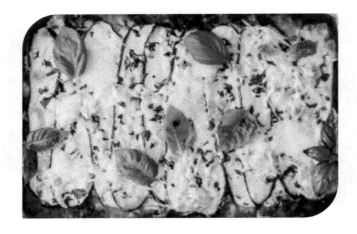

Ingredients

- 1 lb of ground meat
- 1 zucchini
- 2 small tomatoes
- ½ onion
- 1 tbsp minced garlic
- salt to taste
- ½ lb sliced mozzarella
- 2 tbsp grated Parmesan cheese

Steps to Cook

6. Make the Bolognese sauce by adding the minced meat, garlic, salt, onion, and tomato.
7. Cook for about 10 minutes and set aside.
8. Peel and cut the zucchini into strips towards the bottom.
9. The zucchini slices should be as thick as a cookie.
10. Take disposable jars and put a 1cm layer of sauce on the bottom
1. Then top with a layer of zucchini slices and a layer of sliced mozzarella.
2. Repeat the layers in sequence: meat, zucchini and cheese. Sprinkle the grated Parmesan on top. Make another tray the same
3. Preheat the air fryer for 5 minutes at 390°F
4. Bake in the fryer for 10 minutes at 350°F
5. Well, now just enjoy this delicacy.

Nutrition Information

- Calories: 352
- Carbohydrates: 13g
- Fat: 21g
- Protein: 24g
- Sugar: 5g
- Cholesterol: 234m

Margherita Pizza

Servings: 4
Preparation time: 25 minutes
Cook time: 25 minutes

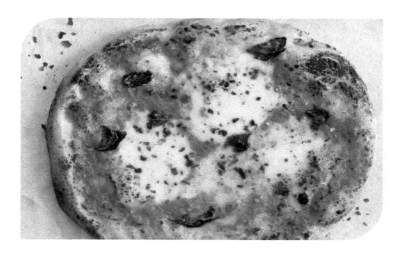

Ingredients

- 10 units of chopped, peeled and peeled tomatoes
- 1 food donation
- 1 tbsp butter
- 1 bunch of fresh basil, to taste
- 1 spoon of sugar
- 2 spoons and olive oil
- 6 slices of bread without peel
- 1 lb grated mozzarella
- Olive oil to taste

Steps to Cook

4. Place the tomatoes in a pan with the butter and 1 sprig of basil and bring to medium heat.
1. Let it cook for 25 minutes, season with salt and sugar. In a baking dish, grease with olive oil, make a layer of bread, put the tomato sauce, the fresh basil leaves, the mozzarella, the basil leaves again, drizzle a little olive oil and finish with a little salt.
2. Place in a preheated air fryer at 350°F for 25 minutes.

Nutrition Information

- Calories: 699
- Carbohydrates: 89.7g
- Fat: 26.8g
- Protein: 32.1g
- Sugar: 7g
- Cholesterol: 17.7mg

Banana Cake

Servings: 2-4
Preparation time: 15 mins
Cook time: 20 minutes

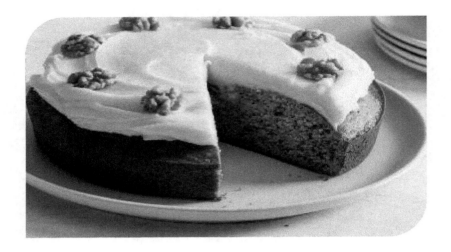

Ingredients

- 2 cups of wheat flour
- ¾ cup sugar
- ½ tbsp baking powder
- ½ tbsp of baking soda
- ½ tbsp of salt
- 6 tbsp soft butter
- 3 eggs
- 1 cup milk
- 1 tbsp of vanilla extract
- 1 cup of chocolate chips
- ½ cup of mashed bananas

Steps to Cook

1. Start greasing a shape that suits your air fryer
2. Whisk the butter and sugar in a large bowl until smooth and fluffy.
3. Then mix the eggs and vanilla and mix well.
4. Now mix the flour, salt, yeast, and baking soda and mix well. Then mix the milk and the banana puree.
5. After everything is mixed, pour the chocolate drops into the dough.
6. Pour the dough into the greased tray and place it in the fryer and bake for 20 minutes at 350°F.

Nutrition Information

- Calories: 323
- Carbohydrates: 61.06g
- Fat: 7.85g
- Protein: 3.74g
- Sugar: 42.66g
- Cholesterol: 32mg

S'mores

Servings: 30
Preparation time: 15 minutes
Cook time: 10 minutes

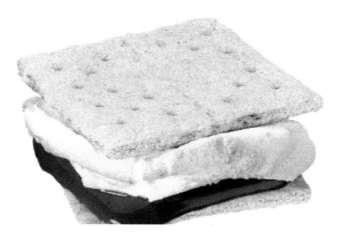

Ingredients

- ½ lb of milk or semi-bitter chocolate
- ½ lb of marshmallow
- Biscuit without filling
- salty like the cream cookie
- Water
- Salt

Steps to Cook

1. You will need a container that can go to the air fryer. Take the container of your choice and place the finely chopped chocolate on the bottom. Make a mixture of milk chocolate with semi-bitter chocolate, however after it was done, since the marshmallow is very sweet.
2. If you are making pillows, divide the chocolate into equal parts for the number of dishes used. Right after you put the chocolate in, overlap them with marshmallows. It is very important that marshmallows are kept well together, with no space between them, so that they do not "fly" through the air fryer. Once done, simply take the dishes to the Air-Fryer for 5 minutes at 350°F.

Nutrition Information

- Calories: 250
- Carbohydrates: 43g
- Fat: 70g
- Protein: 3g
- Sugar: 23g
- Cholesterol: 10mg

Rosca de Polvilho

Servings: 4-6
Preparation time: 5 minutes
Cook time: 30 minutes

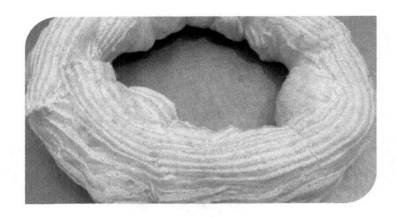

Ingredients

- 2 ¼ lb sour powder
- 3 eggs
- 2 tbsp of margarine
- 1 cup boiling water
- 1 tbsp of salt
- Milk to splash the dough

Steps to Cook

1. In a bowl, place the starch and boiling water for blanching.
2. Reserve the warm milk, and then mix all the ingredients, with the ready mix add the milk to knit in the dough.
3. Form the threads and bake in a hot oven at 480°F for about 30 minutes.

Nutrition Information

- Calories: 214
- Carbohydrates: 29g
- Fat: 9g
- Protein: 2g
- Sugar: 10g
- Cholesterol: 300mg

Banana Covered-Soft Paste

Servings: 2-4
Preparation time: 10 minutes
Cook time: 5 minutes

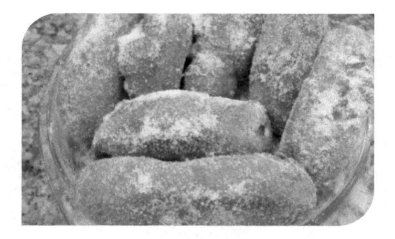

Ingredients

- ½ lb of wheat flour
- 1 cup milk
- 2 eggs
- 3 ½ oz. of sugar
- ½ tbsp of baking powder
- 20 bananas

Steps to Cook

1. Put all the ingredients in a bowl. Stir with a spoon or with your hands until you get a homogeneous mass.
2. Preheat the air fryer at 320°F for a few minutes.
3. Peel the bananas, now with a fork place the banana in the dough until it is completely wrapped. Be careful to put it in the air fryer for 5 minutes to splash after all the fried covered bananas are passed over the cinnamon and sugar. So it only works.

Nutrition Information

- Calories: 107
- Carbohydrates: 19.6g
- Fat: 4.5g
- Protein: 1.3g
- Sugar: 13g
- Cholesterol: 0mg

Coconut Tartlets

Servings: 6
Preparation time: 5 minutes
Cook time: 35 minutes

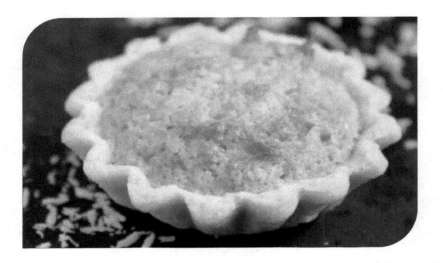

Ingredients

- 1 cup of condensed milk
- 1 cup dry grated coconut
- 2 units of egg
- 10 puff pastry discs
- margarine to grease the pans to taste

Steps to Cook

1. In a bowl, mix the condensed milk, the dried grated coconut and the eggs.
2. Mix well and let stand.
3. On a greased pie with margarine, place a puff pastry disk.
4. Place them on a baking sheet.
5. Place in the air fryer, preheated to 350^0F for 35 minutes until the filling is golden.
6. Remove from the air fryer, let cool, remove from the mold and serve.

Nutrition Information

- Calories: 168
- Carbohydrates: 18g
- Fat: 9.6g
- Protein: 1.7g
- Sugar: 7.7g
- Cholesterol: 0mg

Honey Bread Buns

Servings: 2-4
Preparation time: 5 minutes
Cook time: 25 minutes

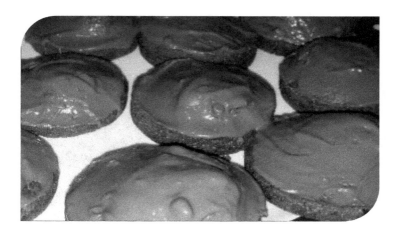

Ingredients

- 1 cup all-purpose flour
- 1 cup milk
- 2 tbsp of honey
- 4 tbsp of sugar
- 2 tbsp of powdered chocolate
- 2 tbsp of oil
- 1 tsp ground cinnamon
- 1 tsp baking soda
- 2 tsp yeast for cakes

Steps to Cook

1. In a refractory container, mix all the cheeses with the cream, arrange them well, and then place them in the Air Fryer basket.
2. Program the Air Fryer for 25 minutes at 320°F or 350°F if you want it well gratinated.

Nutrition Information

- Calories: 130
- Carbohydrates: 25g
- Fat: 2g
- Protein: 4g
- Sugar: 4g
- Cholesterol: 0mg

Herbs Bread

Servings: 4
Preparation time: 5 minutes
Cook time: 25 minutes

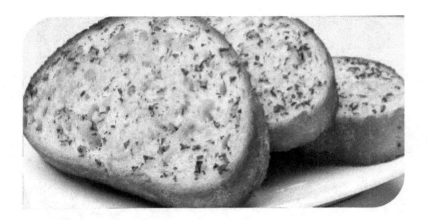

Ingredients

- 1 cup boiling milk
- 3 medium onions
- 1 cup of oil
- 2 tbsp of shallow sugar
- ½ sprig of parsley and chives
- 2 tbsp of oregano
- 1 bunch of basil
- 3 garlic cloves
- 3 whole eggs
- 1 tbsp of salt
- 3 yeast tablets
- 1 beaten egg yolk
- 2 ¼ lbs wheat

Steps to Cook

1. Beat the boiling milk with the onions and add the other ingredients in the order of the recipe one by one and beat, except the wheat.
2. After mixing all the ingredients, pour into a bowl and add the wheat until just right. The dough should be kneaded until it is released from the hands.
3. Let stand until doubled in size (approximately 20 minutes). Then shape the loaves or fill them to taste.
4. Its color will be greenish.
5. Let it sit for a few more minutes.
6. Before roasting, grease lightly beaten egg yolk with 1 tablespoon soy sauce and bake over medium heat until golden brown.
7. It looks super different and smooth.

Nutrition Information

- Calories: 440
- Carbohydrates: 10.5g
- Fat: 21.2g
- Protein: 25.1g
- Sugar: 0g
- Cholesterol: 103mg

Cheesecake

Servings: 2-4
Preparation time: 15 minutes
Cook time: 15 minutes

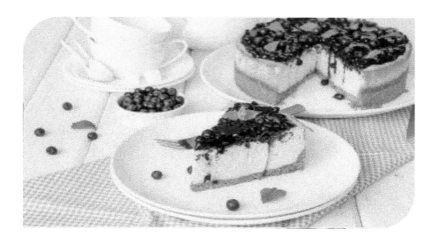

Ingredients

Mass:
- 1 package of cornstarch cookies
- 1 food donation
- 5 tbsp of butter

Filling:
- 1 can of condensed milk
- 7 oz. of cream cheese
- ½ oz. of colorless gelatin without flavor
- 1 can of sour cream
- blackberry jam to taste

Steps to Cook

Mass:
1. Grind the cookies and mix with the butter to form dough.
2. Line a refractory and put in the air fryer at 320°F for 4 to 5 minutes and set aside.

Filling:
3. Beat the condensed milk and cream cheese for 10 minutes.
4. Add the cream and gelatin dissolved in the air fryer for 30 seconds at 400°F.

Topping:
5. Top with jam, unmold, and serve cold.

Nutrition Information

- Calories: 468
- Carbohydrates: 40g
- Fat: 29.5g
- Protein: 7.7g
- Sugar: 25g
- Cholesterol: 76.2mg

Lemon Cake

Servings: 6-8
Preparation time: 30 mins
Cook time: 15 minutes

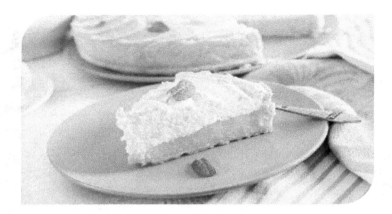

Ingredients

- 4 oz. unsalted butter
- 7 oz. of sugar
- 1 tsp of vanilla essence
- 3 eggs
- 8 oz. flour
- 1 pinch of salt
- 1 tsp baking powder
- ½ cup milk
- To fill and topping:
- 14 oz. condensed milk
- 2 lemons
- 1 box of fresh whipped cream

Steps to Cook

1. In an electric mixer, beat the butter with the sugar until it turns into a cream.
2. Add the lightly beaten eggs with a spoon and the vanilla. Mix well.
3. Gradually add the wheat flour with the yeast and a pinch of salt.
4. Mix everything with a spoon or fuel to avoid damaging your kitchen when using an electric mixer.
5. Beat 10 seconds just to mix a little.
6. Add milk, gradually adding. Beat until well mixed.
7. Great, you already have the perfect dough.
8. You may or may not use silicone-shaped cake paper and place the dough. We did not use it.
9. Put the dough in the molds, but do not overfill it, leave a margin for the cake to grow or it will overflow when baking.
10. Preheat the Air Fryer to 350°F for 3 minutes.
11. Bake 12 to 16 minutes at 350°F. After 10 minutes, check the tip of the cake with a toothpick. Glue half of the dough; if it is dry, the cake is ready.
12. Let's make a cream with the condensed milk and the lemon.

13. Bring condensed milk to heat for 5 minutes. We want a cream.
14. The point is before the harvest point.
15. Then, squeeze 2 lemons and mix well. Let the filling rest.
16. After grilling, allow it to cool slightly to remove from the mold.
17. Slowly remove the cookies from the pan. Whip the whipped cream or fresh cream mixture until it reaches a constant point.

Nutrition Information

- Calories: 421
- Carbohydrates: 65g
- Fat: 16g

- Protein: 4.2g
- Sugar: 47g
- Cholesterol: 74mg

Conclusion

Finally, we have seen a number of advantages to using an air fryer. And the most important of these types of fryers, without a doubt, the ease it offers us to eat delicious food with little fat. By not using oil for frying, you can consume elaborate and much healthier dishes. Your food will retain all its flavor and properties with much less fat than if we cooked them in a normal fryer.

In addition, you have seen how you can prepare countless recipes, many more than in a normal fryer. In oil fryers, many products (such as fish or raw meat) cannot be cooked because they will soak in the oil and become too fatty. However, in the air fryer we do not have that problem.

Enjoy those recipes and we recommend you to follow the proportions proposed in each recipe for an incredible experience.

CPSIA information can be obtained
at www.ICGtesting.com
Printed in the USA
BVHW010946240820
587155BV00016B/136